Walking Portland

A **FALCON** GUIDE®

Walking Portland

Sybilla Avery Cook

 Endorsed by the American Volkssport Association

FALCON GUIDE®

GUILFORD, CONNECTICUT
HELENA, MONTANA
AN IMPRINT OF THE GLOBE PEQUOT PRESS

A FALCON GUIDE®

Falcon and FalconGuide are registered trademarks of Morris Book Publishing, LLC.

Cover photo: Tom McCall Waterfront Park, by Charles A. Blakeslee
All black-and-white photos by Sybilla Avery Cook unless otherwise noted.

Cataloging-in-Publication data is on record at the Library of Congress.

ISBN-13: 978-1-56044-604-0
ISBN-10: 1-56044-604-8

Printed in the United States of America
First Edition/Fifth Printing

To Carolyn and Bob Cook

This couldn't have been written without you.

Contents

the walks

Acknowledgments

This book could not have been written without help from many wonderful people. First and foremost are my son, daughter-in-law, and other family members who provided information, companionship, support, meals, and a place to sleep.

I especially want to thank those who volunteered to read and walk the walks, and then patiently made suggestions and answered questions. These are Brother Gregory OSM, Jan Aust, Liz Bailey, Wendy Bumgardner, Fran Corcoran, Katherine Diack, Grace Mitchell, Hope Hyde, Marianne Kadas, Deanne Kennedy, Eric and Doris Kimmel, Rebecca Macy, Grace Mitchell, Bob Parsons, Ruth Pennington, Jill Schatz, Lisa and Brant Williams. I'm also grateful to Cindy, Sara, Shirley, and other walkers along the way who shared memories, observations, and knowledge.

Mia Matusow of Portland Parks and Recreation and Myrla Magness of the Port of Portland went out of their way to assist me. Diana Anderson and Philip Columbo of the Tri-Met Transit Authority, Linda Anderson of the Mallory Hotel, Mitch Ellovitz of Children's Place Bookstore, Betty Pakenen of RiverPlace Book Merchants, Katrina Gilkey of the Regional Arts and Culture Council, Rosemary White of Lloyd Center, Laura Simon of the Hollywood branch of the Multnomah County Library, Mary Sicilia of Trinity Cathedral, and Jim Stell of the DoubleTree Hotel at Lloyd Center provided descriptions and maps. Pam England of the Portland Oregon Visitors Association, Marilyn O'Grady of Hoyt Arboretum, Rich VanRheen of the Portland Fire Bureau, and Mark Merrill of the Portland Police Bureau were excellent resources, as were Bob Akers, Ted VanVeen, Carol Wild, and Bobbi Wodtli. Debbie Bixby and Jim Long provided personal anecdotes, and Dorothy

Moll, Shirley Buckingham, and Ellen Smith provided willing ears. More information came from Dave Hutchison, Cindy Royce, and Lois Soulia of the Umpqua Community College Library. My husband, John Cook, helped with maps.

Other staff at Independent Living Resources, Portland Parks and Recreation, Oregon Historical Society, Hoyt Arboretum, World Forestry Center, Portland Pioneer Square Association, and Portland Oregon Visitors Association were also helpful.

Finally, I want to thank the countless volunteers of the Portland Audubon Society, Washington Park Hosts, and many of the "Friends" groups, including Crystal Springs Rhododendron Garden, Marquam Park, Powell Butte, Tryon Creek State Park, and others. Portland would not be the wonderful place it is today without them.

Map Legend

Walk Route, paved		Hospital	
Walk Route, unpaved		Tennis Courts	
Interstate Highways		Swimming Pool	
Streets and Roads		Gate	
Hiking/Walking Trail		Overlook	
MAX Light Rail		River or Stream	
Start/Finish of Loop Walk	S/F	Waterfall	
Stairway	or	Lake or Pond	
Parking Area	P	Park or Garden Area	
Building		Interstate	00
Church or Cathedral		U.S. Highway	00
Restrooms, Male and Female		State and County Roads	00
Wheelchair Access		Map Orientation	N
Picnic Area		Scale of Distance	0 0.5 1 Miles
Playground		Point of Interest Key	7

Overview Map

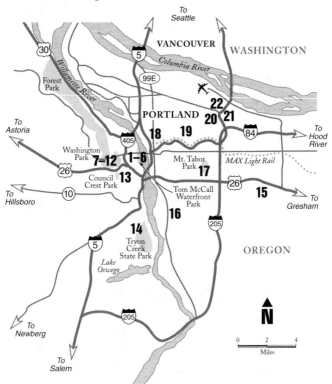

Foreword

For almost twenty years, Falcon Publishing has guided millions of people to America's wild outside, showing them where to paddle, hike, bike, bird, fish, climb, and drive America. With this walking series, we at Falcon ask you to try something even wilder. We invite you to experience this country from its sidewalks, not its back roads, and to stroll through some of America's most interesting cities.

In their haste to get where they are going, travelers often bypass this country's cities, and in the process they miss the historic and scenic treasures hidden among the bricks. Many people seek spectacular scenery and beautiful settings on top of the mountains, along the rivers, and in the woods. While nothing can replace the serenity and inspiration of America's natural wonders, we often overlook the beauty of the American urban landscape.

The steel and glass of a city's municipal mountains reflect the sunlight and make people feel small in the shadows. Birds sing in city parks, water burbles in the fountains, and along the sidewalks walkers can still see abundant wildlife—their fellow human beings.

We hope that Falcon's many outdoor guidebooks have encouraged people not only to explore and enjoy America's natural beauty but also to preserve and protect it. America's cities also are meant to be enjoyed and explored, and their irreplaceable treasures also need care and protection.

So when travelers and walkers want to explore something that is inspirational and beautiful, we hope they will lace up their walking shoes and point their feet toward one of this country's many cities. For there along the walkways, they are sure to discover the excitement, history, beauty, and charm of urban America.—*The Editors*

Preface: Come Walk Portland

Look up, look down, look all around
To see the sights in Portland town.

Each time I walk through Portland, this bit of rhyme runs through my head. Interesting signs, architectural details, and an eclectic assortment of art pieces are on every side, overhead, and underfoot. These unexpected touches are among the amenities that make this such a wonderful place for pedestrians.

Tucked between the Pacific Ocean and the Cascade Range at the confluence of the Columbia and Willamette rivers, Portland delights walkers with its natural beauty. The seafarers and merchants who founded this port city were experienced travelers. Having enjoyed the parks and plazas of the world's loveliest cities, they created a community that included grassy sanctuaries within this City of Roses.

In spite of all the rain jokes, the city's generally mild weather is a boon to walkers. "Rainy" days are often only misty. The sunny summer days are among Portland's best-kept secrets.

Portland was founded in 1845, but fire or flood destroyed most of the early wooden buildings. Elegant and architecturally interesting turn-of-the-century structures replaced them. As you amble through the city, you will pass many graceful old mansions and walk through neighborhoods that embody what was then state-of-the-art planning. Snowcapped Mount Hood and Mount St. Helens form the backdrop to parks, forests, sloughs, the Willamette River waterfront, and Portland's world-famous roses.

Portlanders are well known for their fondness for books, basketball, and brewpubs, so the downtown beckons with good bookstores, a variety of shops, casual eateries, elegant dining, and pubs where you can quench your thirst. Depending upon when you are in town, you may catch one of the many special events held along the restored downtown waterfront or in Civic Stadium, the Coliseum, the Convention Center, and the Rose Garden.

If you are in Portland on business, you will find stress-free getaways within walking distance of your hotel. If you live in Oregon, *Walking Portland* will give you and your visitors a taste of what makes Portland special. From forest trails to waterfront promenades, Portland offers business travelers, tourists, and residents many miles of enjoyable walking.

Introduction

Walking a city's boulevards and avenues can take you into
its heart and give you a feel for its pulse and personality.
Looking up from the sidewalk, you can appreciate a city's
architecture. Peering in from the sidewalk, you can find the
quaint shops, local museums, and great eateries that give a
city its charm and personality. From a city's nature paths,
you can smell the flowers, glimpse the wildlife, gaze at a
lake, or hear a creek gurgle, and only from the sidewalk can
you get close enough to read the historical plaques and watch
the people.

When you walk a city, you get it all: adventure, scenery,
local color, good exercise, and fun.

How to use this guide

We have designed this book so that you can easily find the
walks that match your interests, time, and energy level. The
"Trip Planner" is the first place you should look when
deciding on a walk. This table will give you the basic information—a walk's distance, estimated walking time, and difficulty. The pictures or icons in the table also tell you specific
things about the walk. Here is what those icons mean:

If you like to take pictures, then you will get some
scenic shots or vistas on this walk. Every walk has
something of interest, but this icon tells you that the route
has great views of the city or the surrounding area. Be sure
to bring your camera.

Somewhere along the route you will have the chance
to get food or a beverage. You will have to glance
through the walk description to determine where and what
kind of food and beverages are available. Walks that do not
have the food icon probably are along nature trails or in
noncommercial areas of the city.

During your walk you will have the chance to shop. More detailed descriptions of the types of stores you will find can be found in the actual walk description.

This walk has something kids will enjoy seeing or doing—a park, zoo, museum, or play equipment. In most cases the walks that carry this icon are shorter and follow an easy, fairly level path. You know your young walking companions best. If your children are patient walkers who do not tire easily, then feel free to choose walks that are longer and harder. In fact, depending on a child's age and energy, most children can do any of the walks in this book. The icon only notes those walks we think they will especially enjoy.

Your path will take you primarily through urban areas. Buildings, small city parks, paved paths are what you will see and pass.

You will pass through a large park or walk in a natural setting where you can see and enjoy nature.

The wheelchair icon means that the path is fully accessible and also that it would be an easy walk for anyone pushing a wheelchair or stroller. We have made every attempt to follow a high standard for accessibility. The icon means there are curb cuts or ramps along the entire route, plus a wheelchair-accessible bathroom somewhere along the course. The path is mostly or entirely paved, and ramps and nonpaved surfaces are clearly described. If you use a wheelchair and have the ability to negotiate curbs and dirt paths or to wheel for longer distances and on uneven surfaces, you may want to skim the directions for the walks that do not carry this symbol. You may find other walks you will enjoy. If in doubt, read the full text of the walk or call the contact source for guidance.

(*A note to joggers:* Joggers also can enjoy many of the walks in this book. If you prefer to jog, first look for those walks with an easy rating. These walks most likely are flat and have a paved or smooth surface. If you want something more challenging, read the walk descriptions to see if the harder routes also appeal to you.)

At the start of each walk chapter, you will find more detailed and specific information that describes the route and what you can expect on your walk:

General location: Here you will get the walk's general location in the city or within a specific area.

Special attractions: Look here to find the specific things you will pass. If this walk has museums, historic homes, restaurants, or wildlife, it will be noted here.

Difficulty rating: We have designed or selected walking routes that an ordinary person in reasonable health can complete. The walks are rated easy, moderate, or difficult. The ease or difficulty does not relate to a person's level of physical fitness. A walk rated easy can be completed by an average walker, but that walker may feel tired when he or she has completed the walk and may feel some muscle soreness.

How easy or hard something is depends on each person. But here are some general guidelines of what the ratings mean:

A walk rated as Easy is flat, with few or no hills. Most likely you will be walking on a maintained surface made of concrete, asphalt, wood, or packed dirt. The path will be easy to follow, and you will be only a block or so from a phone, other people, or businesses. If the walk is less than a mile, you may be able to walk comfortably in street shoes.

A walk rated as Moderate includes some hills, and a few may be steep. The path may include stretches of sand, dirt, gravel, or small crushed rock. The path is easy to follow, but you may not always have street or sidewalk signs, so you may have to check your map or directions. You may be as much as half a mile from the nearest business or people. You should wear walking shoes.

A walk rated as Difficult probably has an unpaved path that includes rocks and patches of vegetation. The trail may have steep ups and downs, and you may have to pause now and then to interpret the walk directions against the natural setting. You will have to carry water, and you may be alone for long stretches during the walk. Walking shoes are a must, and hiking boots may be helpful.

Distance: This gives the total distance of the walk in miles.

Estimated time: The time allotted for each walk is based on walking time only, which is calculated at about 30 minutes per mile—a slow pace. Most people have no trouble walking one mile in 30 minutes, and people with some walking experience often walk a 20-minute mile. If the walk includes museums, shops, or restaurants, add sightseeing time to the estimate.

Services: Here you will find out if such things as restrooms, parking, refreshments, or information centers are available and where you are likely to find them.

Restrictions: The most often noted restriction is pets, which almost always have to be leashed in a city. Most cities also have strict "pooper-scooper" laws, and they enforce them. But restrictions may also include the hours or days a museum or business is open, age requirements, or whether you can ride a bike on the path. If there is something you cannot do on this walk, it will be noted here.

For more information: Each walk includes at least one contact source for you to call for more information. If an agency or business is named as a contact, you will find its phone number and address in Appendix B. This appendix also includes contact information for any business or agency mentioned anywhere in the book.

Getting started: Here you will find specific directions to the starting point. Most walks are closed loops, which means they begin and end at the same point. Thus, you do not have to worry about finding your car or your way back to the bus stop when your walk is over.

In those cities with excellent transportation, such as Portland, it may be easy—and sometimes even more interesting—to end a few of your walks away from the starting point. When this happens, you will get clear directions on how to take public transportation back to your starting point.

If a walk is not a closed loop, this section will tell you where the walk ends, and you will find the exact directions back to your starting point at the end of the walk's directions.

Some downtown walks can be started at any one of several hotels the walk passes. The directions will be for the main starting point, but this section will tell you if it is possible to pick up the walk at other locations. If you are staying at a downtown hotel, it is likely that a walk passes in front of or near your hotel's entrance.

Public transportation: Many cities have excellent transportation systems; others have limited services. If it is possible to take a bus or commuter train to the walk's starting point, you will find the bus or train noted here. You may also find some information about where the bus or train stops and how often and when it runs.

Overview: Every part of a city has a story. Here is where you will find the story or stories about the people, neighborhoods, and history connected to your walk.

The walk

When you reach this point, you are ready to start walking. In this section you will find specific and detailed directions, and you will also learn more about the things you pass. Those who want only the directions and none of the extras can find the straightforward directions by looking for the ➤

What to wear

The best advice on what to wear is to wear something comfortable. Leave behind anything that binds, pinches, rides up, falls down, slips off the shoulder, or comes undone. Otherwise, let common sense, the weather, and your own body tell you what to wear.

Your feet take the hardest pounding when you walk, so wear good shoes. Sandals, shoes with noticeable heels, or any shoes you rarely wear are not good choices. Some running shoes make superb walking shoes. Choose running shoes with wide heels, little-to-no narrowing under the arch, noticeable tread designs, and firm insoles.

If you will be walking in the sun, in the heat of the day, in the wind, or along a route with little to no shade, be sure to take along a hat or scarf. Gloves are a must to keep your hands from chapping in the winter, and sunscreen is important year-round.

What to take

Be sure to take water. Strap a bottle to your pack or tuck a small bottle in a pocket. If you are walking several miles with a dog, remember to take a small bowl so that your pet can also have a drink.

Carry some water even if you will be walking where refreshments are available. Several small sips taken through-

6

out a walk are more effective than one large drink at the walk's end. Also avoid drinks with caffeine or alcohol because they deplete rather than replenish your body's fluids.

A fanny pack also comes in handy. It can hold your water, as well as your keys, money, and sunglasses, and leave your hands free to read your directions. If you will be gone for several hours and will walk where there are few or no services, a light backpack can carry beverages and snacks.

Safety and street savvy

Mention a big city and many people immediately think of safety. Some common questions are "Is it safe to walk during the day?" "What about at night?" "What areas should I avoid?"

Safety should be a common-sense concern whether you are walking in a small town or a big city, but safety does not have to be your overriding concern. America's cities are enjoyable places, and if you follow some basic tips, you will find that these cities are also safe places.

Any safety mishap in a large city is likely to come from petty theft and vandalism. So, the biggest tip is simple: do not tempt thieves. Purses dangling on shoulder straps or slung over your arm, wallets peeking out of pockets, arms burdened with packages, valuables on the car seat—all of these things attract the pickpocket, purse snatcher, or thief because you look like someone who could be easily relieved of your possessions.

Do not carry a purse. Put your money in a money belt or tuck your wallet in a deep side pocket of your pants or skirt or in a fanny pack that rides over your hip bone or stomach. Lock your valuables in the trunk of your car before you park and leave for your walk. Protect your camera by wearing the strap across your chest, not just over your shoulder. Better yet, put your camera in a backpack.

Trip Planner

the walks

Walk name	Difficulty	Distance (miles)	Time	🦽	🏙	🌿	🛍	📖	🔍	📷
Downtown										
1. Riverfront and Old Town	easy	3	2 hrs	✓	✓		✓	✓	✓	✓
2. Public Buildings and Portland Center	easy	3.25	2 hrs	✓	✓		✓	✓	✓	
3. South Park Blocks	easy	3.25	1.5 hrs	✓	✓		✓	✓	✓	
4. Chinatown and the Pearl District	easy	3.5	2 hrs	✓	✓		✓	✓	✓	✓
5. Uptown and Nob Hill	easy	4	2.5 hrs		✓		✓	✓	✓	✓
6. Circling Downtown	easy	6.5	4 hrs		✓		✓	✓	✓	✓
West										
7. Audubon House and Bird Sanctuary	moderate	1	1 hr			✓	✓	✓		✓
8. Woods and Gardens Loop	difficult	3.3–8.3	2–6 hrs			✓	✓	✓	✓	✓
9. Vietnam Veterans Memorial and The World Forestry Center	easy	2	1 hr	✓		✓	✓	✓	✓	✓
10. The Hoyt Arboretum Conifer Trail	easy	1	45 min			✓		✓	✓	✓
11. The Hoyt Arboretum Bristlecone Trail	easy	.5	30 min	✓		✓		✓	✓	✓

		Difficulty	Distance (mi)	Time	Wheelchair access	City setting	Nature setting	Good for kids	Shopping	Food	Bring camera
12.	Washington Park	easy	2–3	1–2 hrs			✓	✓	✓	✓	✓
Southwest											
13.	Council Crest	difficult	4.5	3 hrs			✓			✓	✓
14.	Tryon Creek State Park	moderate	3	2 hrs		✓	✓			✓	✓
Southeast											
15.	Powell Butte Nature Park	moderate	3	1.5 hrs		✓	✓	✓		✓	✓
16.	Crystal Springs and Johnson Creek	moderate	2.5	2 hrs			✓	✓		✓	✓
17.	Mount Tabor Park	moderate	2	1 hr			✓	✓		✓	✓
Northeast											
18.	Convention Center and Lloyd Center	easy	4	2 hrs		✓			✓	✓	✓
19.	Beverly Cleary's Neighborhoods	easy	7	4 hrs		✓			✓	✓	✓
20.	The Grotto	easy	1	1 hr		✓			✓	✓	✓
International Airport Area											
21.	Airport Way	easy	1.5	45 min		✓		✓	✓	✓	✓
22.	Alderwood Road	easy	1.5	45 min					✓	✓	✓

9

the icons

Wheelchair access | City setting | Nature setting | Good for kids | Shopping | Food | Bring camera

You also will feel safer if you remember the following:

•Be aware of your surroundings and the people near you.
•Avoid parks or other isolated places at night.
•Walk with others.
•Walk in well-lit and well-traveled areas.
•Stop and ask directions if you get lost.

The walks in this book were selected by people who had safety in mind. No walk will take you through a bad neighborhood or into an area that is known to be dangerous. Relax, and enjoy your walk.

Share the fun

We have tried to walk you to and through the best Portland has to offer. But you surely will discover other wonderful things—a fabulous bakery, a park tucked inside a neighborhood, a historic tidbit, or an interesting museum. Be sure to write us and share your discovery. We would love to hear from you.

Meet Portland

Fast Facts

General

County: Multnomah. Along with Washington and Clackamas counties, these make up the Tri-county region of the Portland metropolitan area. The surrounding counties of Columbia and Yamhill in Oregon, and Washington's Clark County are also part of the metropolitan area.

Time Zone: Pacific
Area Code: 503

Size

Oregon's largest city
471,325 people
1.7 million people in metro area
130 square miles

Geographic location

Elevation: 173 feet above sea level
Latitude: 40 miles east of the West 122nd meridian
Longitude: 30 miles north of the 45th parallel (halfway
mark between the North Pole and the equator)
Miles to the Pacific Ocean: 78
Miles to Mount Hood: 65

Climate

Average yearly precipitation: 37 inches
Average yearly days of sunshine: 66
Average yearly snowfall: seldom more than a couple of
inches per year
Maximum average temperature: 81.6 degrees F
Minimum average temperature: 38.5 degrees F
Average humidity: 60 percent
Average temperatures: 33.5 in January; 79.5 in July.

Getting there

Major highways
Interstates: I-5, I-84, I-205, I-405
U.S. highways: US 30, US 26
State highways: 99E

Airport Service
Most domestic airlines and some international airlines, including Air BC, Alaska, America West, American, Canadian Regional, Continental, Delta, Hawaiian, Horizon Air, Northwest, Reno Air, Southwest, TWA, United, Western Pacific

Bridges
Ten bridges link Portland's east and west sides by carrying pedestrian and auto traffic over the Willamette River. The oldest of these is the Hawthorne Bridge, built in 1910 and the oldest lift bridge in the world. The Hawthorne Bridge will be closed for repairs between March 1998 and March 1999.

Recreation

Golf courses: 13 within city limits, 10 are public. The web pages http://www.services.golfweb.com and http://www.Oregongolf.com give full information on these.

Parks: There are 37,000 acres in more than 200 parks in the metro area.

Boat tours: The *Portland Spirit* is docked at Tom McCall Waterfront Park near the Portland Oregon Visitors Association (POVA) office and offers various sightseeing trips up and down the Willamette River. Phone 1-800-224-3901 for information. The sternwheeler *Cascade Queen* is docked at RiverPlace Marina and offers two-hour narrated cruises of the Portland harbor area. Phone: 503-223-3928.

Major industries

Commercial trade, manufacture of electronic instruments, metal products, machinery, and transportation equipment.

Media

Television stations

ABC—Channel 2

CBS—Channel 6

NBC—Channel 8

PBS—Channel 10

KPTV—Channel 12

Fox—Channel 49

Radio stations

KXL 750 AM—All news and weather

KOPB 91.5 FM—Oregon Public Broadcasting

Newspapers

The *Oregonian*, morning daily

Willamette Week, free weekly tabloid, covers movies, nightclubs, music, art, books, drama, other events

Portland Parent, free monthly tabloid covering recreational activities and area events that are fun for kids

Special annual events

Call 1-800-962-3700 for a visitor's guide, or use the website at http://www.pova.com. Call the Rose Quarter Event Hotline at 503-321-3211 for events at the Rose Garden or Memorial Coliseum.

- April—Tryon Creek State Park Trillium Festival
- June—Portland Rose Festival: a month of events
- July—Oregon Brewers Festival
- July—Waterfront Blues Festival
- July—Multnomah County Fair
- August—The Bite: A Taste of Portland
- September—Horst Mager's Rheinlander Oktoberfest
- October—Portland Marathon

- October—Annual Greek Festival
- October—LitEruption
- December—Christmas Ships: Parade of Lights
- December—Zoolights Festival

In the know

Weather

Portland enjoys a mild climate year-round. July is the warmest month, with an average temperature of 79.5 degrees F. January is the coldest, with an average temperature of 33 degrees F. Few days have measurable snow.

Despite the jokes, the annual rainfall is less than many other major cities. It just falls more often between October and May. An entire day of rainfall may measure less than a quarter inch, so you can generally walk year-round.

Summer days are usually sunny, with low humidity. However nights are generally cool, so bring along a sweater or jacket. Dressing in layers is a good idea year-round.

Transportation

By car: Interstate 5 runs north and south through the city, and Interstate 84 brings in traffic from the east. Most addresses are easy to find, since most avenues are numbered, beginning at the Willamette River. The numbering runs to the west on the west side of the river, and to the east on the east side. The larger the number, the farther away you are from downtown.

Portland is divided into five areas: Northeast, Southeast, Northwest, Southwest, and North. Burnside Street divides the north and south parts of the city, while the Willamette River divides east from west. The north side of the city is north of Interstate 405 and mostly west of Interstate 5. House numbers begin at zero from Burnside, with numbers increasing to the north and to the south.

By bus: Tri-Met is the regional transportation authority, providing 85 convenient and inexpensive bus routes through the region's three counties. Nearly all connect in the downtown transit mall along 5th and 6th Avenues. The buses are free in the downtown's 300-block "Fareless Square."

By train: The MAX light-rail system runs from Pioneer Courthouse Square through the Old Town area of downtown, then east to Lloyd Center and Gresham, and, with line entirely opened by September 1998, west to Hillsboro. Amtrak comes into the city at Union Station in the Old Town/Chinatown neighborhood.

By air: Portland International Airport is on the northeast side of the city along the Columbia River. Buses bring you downtown in less than half an hour.

Safety

The Association for Portland Progress and the City of Portland created the Downtown Clean & Safe Services District in order to make sure the downtown was safe, inviting, and active for businesses, residents, and visitors. Operation of the district is paid for with a business license fee paid by property managers and building owners and provides security, crime prevention, and cleaning services in the 212-block downtown area.

The Portland Guides are one of these innovative services. These guides in kelly-green jackets and caps roam the downtown seven days a week in teams of two. They are trained to offer assistance, answer questions, and make sure visitors feel welcome. Police officers also continually patrol downtown.

Nice evenings and special events always bring people out, and the well-lit areas that are busy with people are generally safe for walkers. Otherwise, as in most cities, it is best to walk during daylight hours.

The Story of Portland

When emigrants on the Oregon Trail reached a fork in the trail, one story says, they had to make a decision about which way to go. One trail was marked with a lump of gold ore. The other had a sign reading, "To Oregon." Those who wanted riches went to California, while those who could read came to Oregon. Despite the implications of this apocryphal story, Oregon attracted entrepreneurs who hoped to make money.

After Lewis and Clark returned from their famous expedition with glowing news of the lands they had discovered, the United States needed an answer to the British settlement at Fort Vancouver. Oregon City, a town at the falls farther up the Willamette River, was founded in 1829 as the first major settlement in Oregon. Francis W. Pettygrove, an employee of a New York City merchant, was sent to Oregon City to open a store. Asa Lovejoy, who originally visited Oregon with missionary Marcus Whitman, saw the town as an ideal place to practice law.

The Clearing

William Overton, the first man to file a land claim on the site that became Portland, was a drifter who was searching for golden opportunities. He staked a claim on a popular camping spot for sailors and traders. It was known as "The Clearing" because over the years the trees had been cut down to feed campfires. Overton offered a half interest in his claim to Lovejoy in return for Lovejoy's filing the claim and paying the 25-cent filing fee. Overton soon decided to move on, and he traded the other half of his claim to Pettygrove in return for $50 worth of supplies.

Another man who was impressed by this clearing was Massachusetts sea captain John H. Couch (pronounced "kooch"), one of the first to bring a ship filled with merchandise up the Willamette River to Oregon City. However, on a subsequent trip, he was unable to navigate that far, and he realized that the site of the Lovejoy-Pettygrove claim would make a better port. He then took up a land claim to the north.

Couch, Lovejoy, and Pettygrove were all profit-seeking entrepreneurs. They were also educated men who brought their knowledge of the world to the frontier. Pettygrove, from Maine, had lived in New York City. Lovejoy was educated at colleges in Amherst and Cambridge, Massachusetts, and had visited many of the great cities of the world. The ideas they had about what constituted a proper city helped to give Portland a good start.

Lovejoy and Pettygrove hired surveyor Thomas Brown to lay out "The Clearing" in a 16-block grid of 200-square-foot blocks and 60-foot-wide streets. They numbered the north-south streets, starting at the Willamette. They gave names to the east-west streets. They also dedicated some of the blocks for public use. Pettygrove built a wharf at the foot of what is now Washington Street and began a road up to the farming area known as the Tualatin Plains. At this point, both men thought the town needed a more dignified name. Lovejoy proposed "Boston," while Pettygrove preferred "Portland." The choice was settled with the toss of a copper coin.

Stumptown

Portland has always had a number of affectionate and not-so-affectionate nicknames that reflect the city's development. Even after the town acquired its first official name, it was usually called "Stumptown" because of the numerous stumps left standing in the streets as trees were cut down to supply building materials. Even when whitewashed, the stumps were a traffic hazard.

In 1848, as the town began to prosper, Lovejoy and Pettygrove sold their claims to Daniel Lownsdale and merchant Benjamin Stark. Lawyer William Chapman and builder Stephen Coffin also purchased land in what is now the downtown area. They began clearing the stumps from the streets, and Lownsdale started another road to the Tualatin Valley. Chapman, who had previously tried to start a railroad, joined Coffin in constructing a plank road so that farmers could bring their produce to town more easily.

By 1859, when Oregon became a state, more than 200 buildings filled the Portland streets. Together, Lownsdale, Chapman, Coffin, Stark, and Couch dedicated more land to public use, including 25 blocks for a park boulevard through the center of the city. These blocks, now known as the Park Blocks, are one of Portland's best-loved features.

The River City

By this time, the town was a thriving port. As the Civil War heated up, emigrants from both sides of the controversy poured into Oregon via the Oregon Trail.

Prospectors came and went, leaving the merchants to make good money. The heavy river commerce attracted longshoremen and Chinese dockworkers. Vicious rivalry and competition developed among the steamship companies, until the Oregon Steam Navigation Company monopolized traffic on both the Columbia and Willamette. Later, some rival companies sprang up, and the railroad was finally completed. The town became known for some of its notorious citizens, such as Joseph Kelly, who bragged that he could shanghai a full crew of men for any ship in less than 12 hours. "Sweet Mary" was the madam of a floating bordello that ran up and down the river, avoiding both the law and taxes.

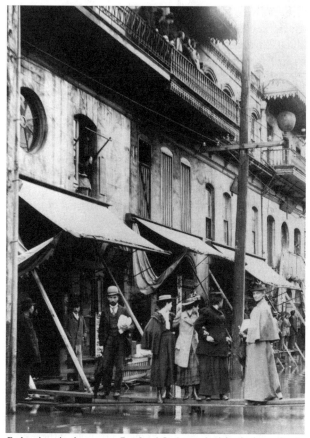

Pedestrians in downtown Portland find travel tricky during a flood in the 1890s. Photo courtesy of Oregon Historical Society 58997

The White City

By the late 1800s, the town had stabilized. The "Great Fire" of 1873 had destroyed all the wooden buildings in 22 downtown blocks, but they had been replaced with more permanent structures, often with cast-iron facades. The completed railroad brought visitors to the city, and a fine hotel became necessary. Railroader Henry Villard hired famous Eastern architect Stanford White to design what became the well-loved Portland Hotel. White's assistant, A. E. Doyle, had been fascinated by the "City Beautiful" ideas displayed at the 1893 World's Fair and Columbian Exposition in Chicago, and he hoped to make Portland a "White City" using terra-cotta trim. Doyle was soon hired by many prospering merchants to implement his ideas, and many of Doyle's buildings still survive.

Seattle had hired the famous landscape firm of the Olmsted brothers to develop their park system. John C. Olmsted, son of the firm's founder, Frederick Olmsted, was sent to the northwest. While here, he was hired to make suggestions for additions and improvements to Portland's city park system. Many of his ideas have slowly been adopted through the years.

The Bridge City

As the city grew on both sides of the Willamette, bridges were needed to connect the two areas. The first bridge was built in 1887, and others soon followed. Today, 10 bridges connect the two sides of the Willamette. Five of these open to allow the passage of river traffic; the others are fixed.

The city east of the river has continued to grow and has conveniently continued the system of numbering all north-south streets. No matter where you are in Portland, it's easy to find your way around.

The City of Roses

The Lewis and Clark Exposition of 1905 brought a great deal of positive attention to Portland, and civic leaders wished to capitalize on the publicity. Since roses were thriving in Portland's gardens—Georgina Pittock staged the first rose show at her home in 1888—Mayor Harry Lane proposed a Festival of Roses to begin in 1907. The International Rose Test Gardens were installed in Washington Park in 1917, and roses have been synonymous with Portland ever since.

The City that Works

This somewhat boastful motto, seen on many municipal vehicles, has some truth to it. Portland has preserved and built on the best of its past. The vision and civic generosity of Portland's founders have enhanced today's city life. Lovejoy's small "dollhouse blocks" make the city a pedestrian's delight. Doyle's "white" buildings light up the downtown.

Today's civic leaders have vision, too. Most older public buildings are surrounded by lawns and fill an entire block. The city code requires newer buildings to include shops and courtyards at sidewalk level. The Metropolitan Art for Public Spaces Act, enacted in 1980, requires that 1 percent of all municipal building costs be allocated to on-site art, and many privately funded buildings have followed suit, so an eclectic assortment of art pieces delights passersby.

The Outdoor City

Today, the "Outdoor City" might be an appropriate nickname for Portland. Its green spaces and sanctuaries didn't just happen. In 1904, the Olmsted brothers visualized a 40-mile loop of parks and boulevards surrounding the city. This vision is slowly being realized in what is still called the "40-Mile Loop," although when completed it will be a 130-mile trail connecting municipal parks with others along the Willamette, Columbia, and Sandy Rivers. Tom McCall Waterfront Park, created by tearing down an expressway, was backed by and named for the former visionary and governor of the same name. Come to Portland and mingle with those who have come to love this city. As you walk, enjoy your surroundings and choose your own nickname for this lovely corner of the Pacific Northwest.

walk 1

Riverfront and Old Town

General location: Downtown Portland, west of Interstate 5.

Special attractions: Historic buildings, interesting shops and restaurants, and the Willamette River waterfront.

Difficulty: Easy, flat, entirely on paved sidewalks with curb cuts.

Distance: 3 miles.

Estimated time: 2 hours.

Services: Restaurants, restrooms, tourist information center.

Restrictions: Days and hours vary at the museums. The Portland Oregon Visitors Association Center is open six days a week, but hours vary. When the center is closed, maps and local information are available in an outside box.

For more information: Contact the Portland Oregon Visitors Association.

Riverfront and Old Town

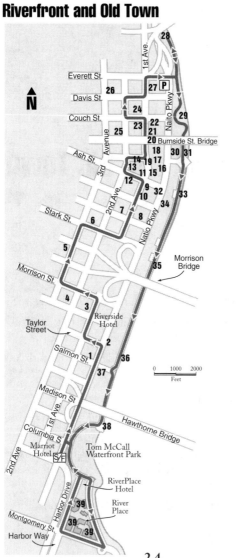

Points of Interest

Getting started: The walk begins at the Marriott Hotel between Clay and Columbia Streets at 1401 SW Naito Parkway. Naito Parkway was formerly named Front Avenue, which is still shown on older maps. From Interstate 5 northbound, exit 299B to Interstate 405, then exit 1A to Naito Parkway. From Interstate 5 southbound take exit 300B, City Center, to the Morrison Bridge, then go south on Naito Parkway to the Marriott.

The "Smart Park" city parking garages provide the most inexpensive parking in Portland. A "Smart Park" is next to the Marriott at 1st Avenue and Jefferson Street. Enter on Jefferson.

Public transportation: All of downtown Portland is within a fareless area—you can ride on a bus anywhere within this area for free. Contact Tri-Met for information about times, fares, and accessibility.

Overview: This riverfront area is where Portland originally was founded and developed. Fires destroyed the first wooden buildings, which were replaced by buildings with cast-iron facades. After major downtown flooding in the late 1800s, businesses moved back from the river leaving these buildings behind. Many old structures were demolished. Those remaining are now being renovated, restored, and reused by tempting shops and restaurants.

An expressway along the riverbank was torn down to create Tom McCall Waterfront Park. Today this entrance to the city hosts many civic and cultural events. It is always full of walkers, cyclers, runners, and people just admiring the view.

The walk

➤Begin at the front door of the Marriott Hotel.

➤Turn left and walk four blocks north to the World Trade Center buildings.

➤Pass the first Trade Center building and cross Salmon Street. The Portland Oregon Visitors Association is currently in this second building but plans to move to Pioneer Courthouse Square in 1999. Volunteers at the visitor center can provide maps and literature, answer all questions, and point out interesting items in the Made in Oregon shop.

➤Continue past the center to Taylor Street. Cross Taylor. A plaque at this corner tells about tiny Mill Ends Park, located in the Naito Parkway traffic island. Dick Fagan, a newspaper columnist, grew tired of seeing an empty hole beneath his office window. He filled it with flowers and later wrote columns about an imaginary leprechaun inhabitant. It became an official city park after Fagan's death.

➤Cross to the traffic island to see this world's smallest park, then return to this corner.

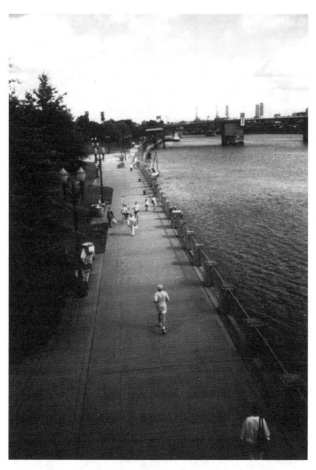

The walk along the Willamette River in Tom McCall Waterfront Park. PHOTO BY ROBERT S. COOK

➤Go straight west on Taylor to 1st Avenue. You are now in the Yamhill Historic District.

➤Turn right and proceed one block to Yamhill.

➤Cross Yamhill and continue to Morrison Street. Across 1st is the Willamette Block Building, one example of the Italianate cast-iron buildings for which this district is noted.

➤Turn left at Morrison Street, cross 1st, and go west to 2nd Avenue.

➤Cross 2nd. The Centennial Block on your left is another example of a cast-iron building.

➤Continue to 3rd Avenue.

➤Turn right at 3rd, cross Morrison, and continue north for two blocks to Washington Street. Notice the Romanesque-style Dekum Building across 3rd. Frank Dekum left the California goldfields with only $2 in his pocket but made a Portland fortune in merchandising and banking. Only local materials were used for this substantial-looking building. A king's head and carved griffins adorn the massive doorway arch, and the lower three stories are faced with sandstone. The upper red-brick stories are decorated with terra-cotta garlands.

➤Cross Washington and proceed north one block.

➤Turn right at the corner of 3rd Avenue and Stark Street. The slender Gothic-style Bishop's House is across Stark. This building, originally constructed in 1879 as an addition to a Roman Catholic cathedral that once stood next door, was restored in 1965. It now houses a restaurant.

➤Proceed east for two blocks to 1st Avenue.

➤Turn left at 1st. Cross Stark and then cross Oak Street. You have entered the Skidmore Historic District, usually referred to as "Old Town." The first building on your left is the 1886 Failing Building, built in a French and Italian style of architecture. Across the street on your right is the 1859 Dielschneider Building, one of the oldest buildings in Portland.

➤Go one block north and cross Pine. Though built within a few years of each other, two very different buildings fill the block's east side between Pine and Ash. The classic red brick 1872 Railway Equipment Company Building with white terra-cotta ornamentation contrasts with the sober, gray, 1876 Scottish Bank Building ornamented only by Scotch thistles.

➤Continue to Ash Street and cross with the light. In the 1880s, the steamship docks were at the river end of Ash, making this a bustling mixed neighborhood of businesses, shipping, and residences.

➤Turn left for one block to 2nd Avenue, passing by the 1871 Poppleton Building. On the southeast corner of Ash and 2nd is the 1889 Glisan Building. This last cast-iron building built in Portland displays a mixture of Romanesque, Gothic, classical, and art nouveau styles.

➤Turn right on 2nd. The 1872 New Market Building on your right originally had a produce market on the first floor and a 2,000-seat theater on the second. Now it is occupied by several small shops and eateries.

➤Proceed to the next corner and turn right on Ankeny Street, passing the Ankeny Colonnade, a remnant of a building formerly on this site.

➤Go to 1st Avenue. Use the crosswalk to cross diagonally to the "Ankeny Arcade" wall. This wall, named after Captain Alexander Ankeny, who built several buildings in this area, displays a variety of cast-iron ornaments. A large sign tells how these were salvaged when the original structures were torn down.

➤Follow the wall to your left and around the corner, going by the iron fence on the north wall of the active Central Fire Station. More fragments are here, along with photographs of the original buildings.

The Jeff Morris Fire Museum can be seen through the large glass windows on the east end of this wall. It is a window museum only, not open to visitors. If you are interested in getting a better view, the firefighters at the station will open the metal gate and let you peer through the north windows within the fence. A 1911 American LaFrance horse-drawn steamer with paint and gold-leaf trim by Mitch Kim is thought to be one of the finest in the world. Most of these fire engines were lovingly restored by Portland firefighters Al Carocci and Frank Maas. The antique ladder truck is pulled by firefighters each June in the annual Rose Festival Starlight Parade.

Many old helmets hang from the ceiling. The switchboard along the back wall dates from the days of horse-drawn engines and was used until 1980. Originally, the ticker tape made a pattern of clicks designating the particular company assigned to a fire. When the horses heard their own particular click pattern, they would move to stand underneath their individual harnesses and wait for them to be dropped from the ceiling.

As you turn from the windows, you will see you are on the south side of a large courtyard, Ankeny Square. Across the square is the Packer-Scott Building, a former warehouse still in commercial use.

From Burnside north, this area of Old Town contains a diverse mixture of artists, crafters, seniors, businesspeople, and those living on the street for a variety of reasons. The sight of some of the "street people" makes some tourists uncomfortable, especially when they are asked to give money.

of interest

The Skidmore Fountain

Stephen Skidmore, founder of a major "pharmaceutical emporium," was a prominent member of Portland society in 1870. Fountains he saw during a European tour impressed him so much that he left a bequest for one to be built here in Portland. He stipulated that it provide water "for horses, men, and dogs."

Colonel Charles Erskine Wood—soldier, lawyer, poet, artist, and lifelong friend of Chief Joseph—knew many people associated with the Eastern art establishment. Appointed to carry out the bequest, he chose the famous New York sculptor Olin Warner. Warner's wife supposedly modeled for one of the supporting bronze caryatids. Wood added the motto, "Good citizens are the riches of a city."

The fountain was shipped from New York City by rail and installed in this central location in 1888. Some Portland citizens—and even a New York newspaper—complained that the creation was too artistic for upstart Portland. Can you imagine what the critics would have said if brewer Henry Weinhard's offer to pipe in beer to the fountain had been accepted?

The Burnside Street Bridge covers 1st Avenue immediately north of the fountain. This covered area combines with Ankeny Park to become Saturday Market, open weekends from March through Christmas Eve. A colorful and eclectic group of 400 artists, artisans, plant growers, and food vendors offers unique handmade items for sale in this, the largest open-air crafts market in the country. All crafts are juried to meet the market's standards.■

The local merchants work hard to keep the area free from trouble, and the district is considered safe for tourists.

The arched colonnades on two sides of the square have different facades, one of which came from an 1883 building on this site. The arches make a marvelous frame for photographs. Go to the one on your left to view the antique Skidmore Fountain.

➤Walk to the Skidmore Fountain.

➤Walk north under the Burnside Bridge. Pass the Skidmore Building, where Stephen Skidmore was born.

➤Continue north to Couch Street past the Blagen Block Building—the last remaining Italianate "commercial palace."

➤Turn left and cross 1st Avenue to the Norton House, once a hotel where President Ulysses S. Grant stayed briefly. You will notice from the signs that you are now in the Couch (pronounced "kooch") District.

➤Cross Couch and proceed west to 2nd Avenue. You are passing the 1906 Fleischner-Mayer Building, once a dry-goods store. This was one of the first buildings restored by the Naito brothers, members of the Japanese-American family that began this area's rejuvenation. Today, the district is filled with art galleries, shops, and restaurants and is a center of Portland nightlife.

➤Stop at the corner of Couch and 2nd. Look diagonally across to see Erickson's Saloon at the southwest corner. Loggers and sailors once frequented its 672-foot-long bar, and, supposedly, many drunk unfortunates were shanghaied from here.

➤Turn right on 2nd to Davis. Turn right again on Davis. As you pass the parking lot on your right, look for the painted butterfly on the back wall of the Fleischner-Mayer Building.

of interest

Captain John Couch

This Couch District is the original land claim of John Couch, a sea captain from Newburyport, Massachusetts. Captain Couch came up the Columbia River in 1840 and decided that Portland would make a good seaport. Since he had spent his maritime career sailing by the North Star, he laid out his claim on true north.

Surveyor Thomas Brown had used a compass in 1845 to lay out the city, and his north-south streets conveniently paralleled the river. However, in Portland, magnetic north deviates 21 degrees east from geographic or true north. The mismatch between the streets north and south of Burnside creates several rhomboid or triangular blocks where some streets merge with others.

The northwest side of town, including the Couch District, is sometimes referred to as the "Alphabet District." Captain Couch must have been a methodical man. He kept the existing system for the north-south avenues—1st, 2nd, and so forth—but chose to name his east-west streets with letters of the alphabet—A, B, C, etc. Later, citizens replaced these with the names of noted Portlanders, but kept the alphabetical order.■

►Turn left at 1st. The parking garage on the northeast corner, trimmed with a neon and aluminum design by David Kerner, has a heliport on the roof.

►Proceed north to Everett. Turn right and cross 1st Avenue at the light. Continue past the parking garage to Naito Parkway, formerly known as Front Avenue. Front was the first paved street in Portland and the site of the first school. It seems fitting that this old street, now a pleasant

of interest

William Sumio Naito (1925-1996)

Bill Naito was a native Portlander and the son of Japanese immigrants Hide and Fukieye Naito. When World War II began, Congress passed the Wartime Relocation Act, forcing all Japanese-American citizens living on the West Coast to move to internment camps. Naito's family chose instead to move in with relatives in Salt Lake City.

As soon as Naito was old enough, he joined the U.S. Army, serving as a translator. After the war he earned degrees in economics from Reed College and the University of Chicago before returning to Portland to join his brother Sam in the family import business.

When the Naito brothers moved their business to Couch Street, they painted the butterfly on the blank wall of the Fleischner-Mayer Building both to attract attention and to symbolize the area's Japanese heritage. Bill Naito began to buy historic buildings and turn them into commercially successful properties. He converted lower floors of his renovated buildings into small shops and provided low-income housing for neighborhood residents on the upper levels. The butterfly now symbolizes the family's transformation of the seamy "Skid Row" area into the vibrant commercial area of today.

Naito was convinced that Portland was a great city with a great future, and his enthusiasm and creativity are behind many of the buildings seen on these downtown walks. He changed Old Town, donated space for Saturday Market, and began the revival of the downtown core.■

and scenic drive, should be renamed in memory of Portland's successful renovator.

➤Use the push button for the walk signal on the street post to your right. Cross Naito Parkway with the signal.

➤Take the steps down to the promenade along the Willamette River. Those who need a ramp will find one a few yards south of the steps. You are now close to the north end of Tom McCall Waterfront Park, where many of Portland's outdoor activities and festivals take place. Watch out for runners and bicyclists. The green glass towers on the other side of the river belong to the Oregon Convention Center.

➤Turn left onto the riverfront walkway. Go north toward the Steel Bridge and find the Friendship Circle, created to commemorate 30 years of sister-city relations with Sapporo, Japan. The tall steel sculpture in the center electronically emits the sounds of ancient Japanese instruments.

➤Circle around the sculpture and return to the walkway. The Willamette River should now be on your left. This concrete walk continues south through Tom McCall Waterfront Park.

➤Continue on the walk until you come to a stone path leading to the right. Take this into the Japanese American Historical Plaza.

➤Continue along the walkway as you leave the Japanese American Historical Plaza.

➤Go under the Burnside Bridge. You are now in one of the waterfront's latest additions, the Waterfront Park Story Garden. This is designed to encourage the imagination of children. Red granite stones and illustrated paving blocks decorate a maze of paths. A polished, red granite throne sits at

of interest

The Japanese American Historical Plaza

Bill Naito developed this plaza in memory of the many people forced to leave their homes because of their ancestry. It is highlighted by two bronze cylinders, "Songs of Innocence" and "Songs of Experience," carved with sketches of soldiers and civilians.

A signpost display of the Bill of Rights is a reminder of how the forced internment of Japanese-Americans during World War II violated every single article. A nearby plaque displays a recent statement of apology and reparation made by the U.S. Congress.

Fractured pieces of stone are pieced together to form the pavement circle that surrounds a large stone in the center. Names of the different Japanese-American relocation camps are carved on the boulder.

Japanese cherry trees are planted on the berms. Haiku verses inscribed in both Japanese and English on stones along the path express how it feels to be uprooted from one's home.■

one end of this land of story, while a granite hare and tortoise watch benignly from the sides.

➤Enjoy the view of Portland's skyline as you continue southward. Walk by the polished, stainless-steel Sculpture Stage, perfect for impromptu open-air performances.

You can see more Old Town buildings across Naito Parkway on your right. South of the fire station with the Jeff Morris window museum is the Smith Block Building. This contains the Oregon Maritime Museum, where two floors of exhibits and models recreate the history of the maritime industry. It also contains a research library and a museum store. It is open year-round, but days and hours vary. Contact the museum for fees and times.

The museum tickets also give access to the steamer *Portland*, moored along the seawall. This ship became the *Lauren Belle* in the 1994 movie *Maverick*. A navy barge, the *Russell*, is docked in front of the *Portland*.

Look for the smokestack on the right of the walkway. This is from the battleship USS *Oregon*, which saw action in Cuba during the Spanish-American War. The smokestack is now a memorial to the Spanish-American War nurses. A bicentennial time capsule inside the stack is to be opened in 2076.

Look down to see markers incised in the pavement that locate early sites in Portland history. A marker for "Indian Camps, 1845" is shortly followed by one for "The Clearing, 1840." A picture shows this place at the time of Portland's founding.

A little farther south are pavement markers for the first wharf built in 1846 and for the Stephens family, whose land claim was across the river. The next marker designates the 1845 townsite. The Lownsdale land claim marker is at Morrison Street.

The docking site for the sternwheeler *Columbia Gorge* is situated just before the Morrison Bridge. This was the first bridge built over the Willamette River. The *Portland Spirit* docking site is on the bridge's other side. Both ships offer river cruises. Beyond the *Spirit*, a brass plaque shows the distances to various Portland bridges.

➤Continue to the Salmon Street Springs fountain. An underground computer changes the spray patterns of the 185 jets every ten minutes.

➤Follow the walkway under the Hawthorne Bridge. Across the river is the red brick tower at OMSI—the Oregon Museum of Science and Industry.

Signs at the little plaza here tell about the Willamette River cleanup under former governor Tom McCall's leadership. They also explain how a six-lane expressway was torn down in 1974 to create this park.

►Continue on the walkway as it arches around to the RiverPlace Hotel, goes past the circle of flags, and heads south. The sternwheeler *Willamette Star* docks at this marina and offers river cruises. You will sometimes see Japanese dragon boats practicing for the annual Rose Festival.

The RiverPlace development has numerous inviting shops and tempting restaurants. Although the shops seem to end at Montgomery Street, there are more around the bend to your right.

►Turn right at Montgomery and go west to Harbor Way. On your left is the RiverPlace Athletic Club.

►Take Harbor Way north to the front of the RiverPlace Hotel.

►Go to the waterfront walkway, retracing your steps back to the crosswalk at Columbia Street.

►Cross Naito Parkway at the traffic signal. You are now at your starting point, the front entrance to the Marriott Hotel.

walk 2

Public Buildings and Portland Center

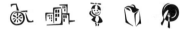

General location: The center of downtown Portland, west of Interstate 5.

Special attractions: Government buildings dating from 1869 through 1997, a variety of fountains, old and new parks, a planned integrated area of shops, offices, and apartments.

Difficulty rating: Easy, flat, entirely on paved sidewalk with curb cuts.

Distance: 3.25 miles.

Estimated time: 2 hours.

Services: Restrooms are available at the Tri-Met offices in Pioneer Courthouse Square and in all public buildings. Most

Public Buildings and Portland Center

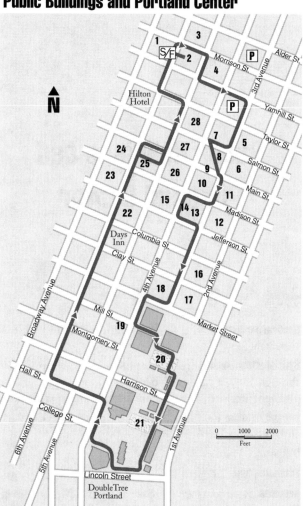

Points of Interest

1 Pioneer Courthouse Square	**15** Portland City Hall
2 Pioneer Courthouse	**16** KOIN Center
3 Meier and Frank Department Store	**17** Portland Civic Auditorium
4 Pioneer Place	**18** Ira Keller Memorial Fountain
5 Auditorium Building	**19** Church of Saint Michael the
6 Mark O. Hatfield Federal Courthouse	Archangel
7 Oregon Sports Hall of Fame Museum	**20** Pettygrove Park
8 Lownsdale Square	**21** Lovejoy Park
9 Elk Fountain	**22** Hoffman Columbia Plaza
10 Chapman Square	**23** University Club
11 Justice Center	**24** Gus Solomon U.S. Courthouse
12 Wyatt/Green Federal Building	**25** Standard Insurance Plaza
13 Terry Schrunk Plaza	**26** Portland Building and *Portlandia*
14 Liberty Bell	**27** Multnomah County Courthouse
	28 Standard Insurance Building

public buildings are open weekdays from 9 A.M. to 5 P.M. Stores and restaurants are located throughout the area.

Restrictions: The Tri-Met information center and the offices of the Pioneer Courthouse Square Association are open Monday through Friday from 8 A.M. to 5 P.M. The restrooms are open everyday from 8 A.M. to 7 P.M. The Police Museum is open Monday through Thursday from 10 A.M. to 3 P.M.

For more information: Contact the Pioneer Courthouse Square Association or the Portland Oregon Visitors Association.

Getting started: This walk begins at Pioneer Courthouse Square, between Broadway and 6th Avenues and Yamhill and Morrison Streets. From Interstate 5 northbound, take the exit to Interstate 405, then take the 6th Avenue exit and continue south to Yamhill Street and Pioneer Courthouse Square. From U.S. Highway 26, take the Market Street exit and follow the City Center signs to 10th Avenue. Turn left on 10th, cross Taylor Street, and turn right on Yamhill for three blocks.

The "Smart Park" city parking garages provide the most inexpensive parking in Portland. There are three in the immediate vicinity. One is on 10th between Yamhill and

Morrison, with an entrance on 10th; one is at 3rd Avenue and Alder Street, with entrances on 3rd and 4th; and one is at 4th Avenue and Yamhill, with the entrance on 4th.

Public transportation: Buses and MAX light-rail lines meet at Pioneer Courthouse Square. The Tri-Met information station and ticket office is situated below the coffee shop and is open Monday through Friday from 8 A.M. to 5 P.M. You can ride anywhere within downtown Portland for free. Contact Tri-Met for information about fares and schedules.

Overview: This walk begins at Portland's Pioneer Courthouse Square, center of today's downtown Portland and easily reached on foot from most downtown hotels. This square, scene of countless festivals and outdoor exhibits, is bordered by department stores, "vertical malls" of specialty shops within reconstructed buildings, excellent restaurants, and one-of-a-kind boutiques.

You will see Portland's oldest courthouse as well as the newest. The Mark O. Hatfield Federal Courthouse was completed in 1997. The walk continues through Portland Center, an area of integrated housing, shops, and offices often called "New Town" or the "Superblocks."

of interest

Pioneer Courthouse Square

Portland's first schoolhouse once stood in this central city block. It was later replaced by the grand and well-loved Portland Hotel, site of many civic and social functions. The hotel was demolished after World War II to make room for the May Company's two-level parking lot, which served the Meier and Frank Department Store.

When the rejuvenated downtown needed a focal point, the May Company not only sold the property to the city but gave half a million dollars toward the square's reconstruction. The square is now managed by the nonprofit Pioneer Courthouse Square Association.

Willard K. Martin, a local architect, won the competition for a "distinctive, dynamic, elegant, and inviting" design. He based his winning plan on European plazas and used Portland's traditional building materials for such classical components as the cast-iron pergola and terra-cotta columns with rose-adorned capitals. Many small artistic touches add interest, such as gargoyles on the water troughs, roses in the bench supports, and history tiles around the small amphitheater. Members of the public bought the bricks used to pave the square, and these are inscribed with their names. There are two amphitheaters, and there is an echo center in the smaller.

The square is where buses, trolleys, and the MAX light-rail system meet. The Tri-Met ticket station is on the plaza level, where helpful people can answer almost every transportation question. You can also purchase tickets at a machine. Walk between pink granite walls flowing with water to find the station or the restrooms.

Powell's Travel Bookstore is under the ramp at the southeastern corner of the square. A Starbucks at the northwest corner offers coffee and snacks. Flowers are sold outside. Wide steps around the plaza provide places to sit, meet a friend, admire the art pieces, read, eat, listen to musicians and the sound of fountains, and watch a fascinating parade of people.

If you're here at noon, keep your eyes and ears open for the day's forecast from the "Weather Machine." Lights flash and a musical fanfare plays as the symbol for the day's weather pops out from the top of the 25-foot column. A sun symbol forecasts a clear day, while a dragon indicates storms. If the blue heron—Portland's city bird—pops out, grab your umbrella or take shelter under the one held by the life-sized sculpture entitled *Allow Me*.

Running Horses, a metal sculpture, is on the Pioneer Courthouse side of the square. Tom Hardy, a noted Oregon artist, has been designing motion-filled sculptures of stone, welded steel, and bronze for more than 50 years. Portland contains many of his birds and other animal pieces. His work can be seen all over the United States; an eagle medallion he created adorns the Franklin Delano Roosevelt Memorial in Washington, D.C. The wrought-iron gate from the former Portland Hotel is nearby, returned to its original location on 6th Avenue.■

The walk

➤Begin the walk on 6th Avenue at the exit between the *Running Horses* statue and the gate from the former Portland Hotel. Stop to look at the milepost sign. It points outs the direction and mileage to many places in Oregon and the world, including Portland's nine sister cities: Ashkelon, Israel; Corinto, Nicaragua; Guadalajara, Mexico; Kaosiung Municipality, China; Suzhou, China; Khabarovsk, Russia; Mutare, Zimbabwe; Sapporo, Japan; and Ulsan, Korea.

➤Cross 6th Avenue to the original Pioneer Courthouse built in 1869. The building's entrance ramp is to the right of the steps.

➤Exit Pioneer Courthouse and turn right onto Morrison Street. Directly across Morrison is the 1909 Meier and Frank Department Store, listed in the National Register of Historic Places. Inside, current merchandise is displayed against a background of original woodwork, bronze elevator doors, and white floor tiles.

of interest

The Pioneer Courthouse

The courthouse was built after the Civil War, and its cupola was the highest structure in town at the time. After another courthouse was built in 1933, plans were made to raze this one. The Oregon Historical Society led a determined fight to save it, and it was finally restored in 1971. Now it is the headquarters of the U.S. Court of Appeals. The lobby is used as a post office.

As you enter the lobby, notice the large cedar figures on either side. Carved in Denmark for the Jacob Kamm Building, they were rescued when that building was demolished and later installed here. The post-office lobby still displays the original woodwork. Along the back wall are pictures showing the building's history.■

This is a good example of architect A. E. Doyle's white-glazed, terra-cotta buildings. He drew his inspiration from the "City Beautiful" display of white Roman- and Renaissance-style buildings at the 1893 World's Fair and Columbian Exposition.

The department store has a variety of decorative designs on its facade. The ornamentation on these terra-cotta buildings was made by hand pressing clay into plaster molds. Look for these details as you tour the city; they are easy to miss because most are above windows and along rooflines.

➤Continue past Pioneer Courthouse to 5th Avenue. Along the sidewalk are Georgia Gerbers's frolicsome *Animals in Pools*. Also referred to as "The Bronze Zoo," these sculptures appeal to animal lovers of all ages. More bronze animals are on the other side of the courthouse.

Portland's entire downtown area is home to an interesting collection of outdoor art. In 1975, the state legislature

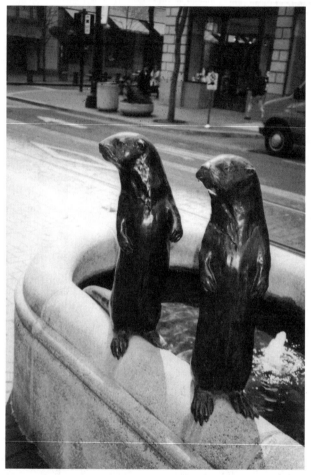

Animals in Pools—Otters. Sculpture by Georgia Gerber.

passed a "1 percent for art" program, allocating this amount of state building-construction money for "publicly accessible works of art." Many of these pieces are located along the 5th and 6th Avenues transit malls.

➤Cross 5th Avenue. Turn right and walk past Pioneer Place. This "vertical mall" contains four levels of intriguing shops. A pathway of blue marbles on the bottom level winds like a river through the shops and food court to a fountain of real water. There is underground access to the parking garage at the corner of 4th and Yamhill.

➤Cross Yamhill. There are four large *Soaring Stones* rising from the sidewalk ahead on 5th. Before reaching them, turn left onto Yamhill.

➤Go to 4th Avenue. Note the plaques enlivening the blank wall on your right. These explain the city symbols: the early symbol of commerce; its transformation into a new symbol, the *Portlandia* sculpture; and the rose from which the city takes its nickname.

➤Cross 4th and proceed to 3rd. At your feet is *Streetwise*, a work of sidewalk art designed by Portland author Katherine Dunn and artist Bill Will. Quotations from people such as Groucho Marx, Anatole France, Ursula Le Guin, Chief Joseph, and "Anonymous" are engraved on granite pavement blocks.

After reading the pavement blocks, study the facade of the parking garage to see the expressive terra-cotta faces. Look across the parking lot on the other side of Yamhill to see a colorful school of aluminum fish swimming *Upstream Downtown* in the openings of the Alder Street parking garage.

➤Turn right on 3rd and continue to Taylor. Across the street is the Auditorium Building, designed by architect Louis

Sullivan. He began the "form follows function" movement, and this is an excellent example of his "Roman column" design. The lower floors make the base, the middle represents the column, and the upper stories are the capitals.

➤Continue to Salmon Street.

➤Turn right onto Salmon, passing the new State of Oregon Sports Hall of Fame museum. This is dedicated to all athletes who ever lived or played in Oregon. The many interactive exhibits include a "virtual-reality" catcher that lets you feel the impact of a 90-mile-an-hour baseball on your glove. Contact the museum for information on hours and prices.

➤Cross Salmon to Lownsdale Square. Take the path diagonally to your left into the center of the square. Lownsdale and Chapman Squares were planned in 1852. In the 1920s, a law was passed designating Lownsdale for men only and Chapman for women.

Lownsdale Square is now the site of a statue erected in 1945 in memory of the men of the Second Oregon Regiment who died during the Spanish-American War. The howitzers at the base were used to defend Fort Sumter at the beginning of the Civil War. A drinking fountain on the west edge of the park is another memorial to Spanish-American volunteers.

➤Continue on this diagonal path to the corner of 3rd and Main. To your right, you can see a large bronze elk on the Main Street traffic island. A drinking trough for horses surrounds the base. Former mayor David Thompson gave this to the city in 1900, and it commemorates a real elk that grazed here regularly in Portland's early days.

➤Cross 3rd. The 1997 Mark O. Hatfield Federal Courthouse sits on this corner. This is the first U.S. courthouse not built on a symmetrical plan. Different facades on the surrounding streets make it appear to be three separate buildings.

If you have time, enter the building. You will have to leave your camera or video recorder with the security guards before taking the elevator to the rooftop garden on the ninth floor. This has a great view of the city and Willamette River. Here are Tom Otterness's delightful and whimsical set of small bronze animal figures portraying different aspects of justice—the *Law of Nature*.

►Turn right and cross Main to the Justice Center. The portico is flanked by travertine sculptures and an arched stained-glass window wall is above the door. The building's wheelchair ramp is at the Madison Street side.

Go into the portico to look at the ceiling. It is covered with a beautiful mosaic of Venetian and fused glass tiles and is lit by hanging lamps resembling copper kettledrums.

More public art is inside the building. The Portland Police Museum is on the sixteenth floor. Admission is free. Contact the museum about hours.

►Leave the Justice Center portico and turn left. Go south to Madison Street. Cross. The building you see here is the Wendall Wyatt/Edith Green Federal Building, named for two former members of the U.S. House of Representatives. Edith Green was Oregon's first congresswoman.

►Turn right, cross 3rd, and continue west to 4th Avenue. You are passing Terry Schrunk Plaza. Its steps and ledges provide pleasant places to sit in the shade of tall trees. Chapman Square is across Madison on your right.

►Turn left onto 4th. On the other side of 4th is the original Portland City Hall, renovated in 1998. A replica of the Liberty

Bell is in the middle of this block on the left. Many photographs, paintings, tiles, and sculptures can be found inside. Architects William Whidden and Ion Lewis designed this sandstone building in 1895, using the classical Roman style of balustrades, Tuscan columns, and a large rotunda. The building is quite a contrast to the teal, postmodern Portland Building across the street!

➤Go to Jefferson Street, turn left, and return to 3rd.

➤Turn right onto 3rd. Go straight to Columbia Street. Cross. The KOIN Center occupies the entire block on the other side of the street. This red-brick tower is shaped like a fat kindergarten crayon with a big blue point. The KOIN television station and other offices are on the lower floors, while luxury apartments fill the upper levels.

➤Continue south, crossing Clay Street. Across 3rd is Portland Civic Auditorium, home of the Portland Opera and Oregon Ballet Theatre. On your right is the Ira Keller Memorial Fountain, a favorite summer play place for Portland youngsters. The shady ponds and splash areas on the upper concrete terraces, together with cascading waterfalls pooling around the stepping stones at the lower level, represent mountains, streams, and other kinds of moving water. "Ira's Fountain" is the highest manmade waterfall in Oregon.

➤Turn right at the walkway on the south side of the fountain. Follow the walkway west to 4th Avenue.

➤Turn left and cross Market Street. Continue south past the telephone building and stop at the Mill Street sign. This is the west edge of the Portland Center urban-renewal project. Thirty-six blocks were razed in the 1950s to create this "New Town" of office buildings, parks, and high-rise apartments. Some streets were turned into pedestrian walkways. Mill Street is one of these.

Diagonally across 4th is the Church of Saint Michael the Archangel. Originally a German cathedral, it later became the Italian National Church and is now a neighborhood Roman Catholic church.

➤Turn left onto the Mill Street walkway and go to the T intersection at the wall adorned with a yellow metal sculpture appropriately named *Awning*. Turn right here and take the first walkway on your left into small Pettygrove Park. Trees and grassy mounds make the park seem larger than it actually is.

➤Continue along the walkway. Take the path on your right to *The Dreamer*, a large golden bronze sculpture filled with urethane foam. When it rains, the foam softens the sound of the raindrops hitting the statue. It is surrounded by a pool.

➤Pass *The Dreamer* and go to the walkway.

➤Turn right and go south on the walkway between highrise apartments and office buildings. Wooden posts mark the location of Harrison Street.

➤Cross Harrison between these posts and continue south until you see another small park on your right. This park, named for Asa Lovejoy, contains a picnic pavilion, concrete terraces, small pools, and a fountain. Author Terence O'Donnell has described this park as "an origami in concrete."

➤Continue on the walkway past the park. Go straight until you spot the small brick fountain known as "The Chimney."

➤Pass the fountain, go to Lincoln Street, and turn right. The DoubleTree Portland is across Lincoln.

➤Turn right onto the next walkway.

➤Follow the walkway to the left to 4th Avenue.

➤Turn right on 4th and walk to the traffic signal at Hall Street.

➤Turn left, cross 4th, and go west two blocks to 6th Avenue.

➤Turn to your right, crossing Hall Street. The Portland State University Bookstore is on the northeast corner of Hall and 6th. Other PSU buildings are across 6th.

➤Continue north on 6th for six blocks until you reach and cross Columbia Street. The next block is filled by the Hoffman Columbia Plaza, another landmark design by Pietro Belluschi.

➤Cross Jefferson. As you walk north, look across 6th Avenue to view the University Club. The Jacobean-style facade resembles college buildings across the country.

➤Continue north and cross Madison Street. The Gus Solomon U.S. Courthouse is directly across the street on your left. The Standard Insurance Plaza fills the block on your right. In front of this building is *The Ring of Time*, a rough metal sculpture shaped like a giant Mobius strip.

➤If the Standard Insurance Plaza is *not* open, go straight ahead to Main Street and turn right. Turn again to your right on 5th Avenue and go to the wide plaza in front of the building.

If the Standard Insurance building *is* open, turn right, cross the small bridge, and enter the front lobby. Go through the glass doors to the 5th Avenue side. Here, you'll get a spectacular view of the Portland Building and *Portlandia*. You are almost on the same level as the statue. Escalators in this area will take you down to 5th Avenue.

Michael Graves's postmodern Portland Building on the other side of 5th Avenue has been controversial since its construction in 1982. The teal-colored tiles and decorative accents give it the appearance of a giant birthday present rather than a city-government office building.

The 38-foot figure of *Portlandia* is made of hammered copper sheeting over a steel armature—the same method used in the *Statue of Liberty*. Her image was adapted from an old Portland city seal.

►Leave the lobby by taking the escalator down to street level, exiting to the 5th Avenue plaza. From this plaza, you will get another view of *Portlandia*. A sign displays a verse from the prize-winning "Ode to Portlandia," as well as some of the statue's statistics and history. At the northeast corner of the Portland Building across the street is a carved stone sculpture, *Interlocking Forms*.

►Go to Main Street. Cross and continue toward Salmon. Look to your right across 5th. The limestone building with terra-cotta decorations is the Multnomah County Courthouse, listed in the National Register of Historic Places.

►Cross Salmon. Continue straight to Taylor Street. Across 5th Avenue to your right is a large marble fountain. Officially entitled *The Quest*, it is sometimes referred to as "Three Groins in the Fountain."

►Turn left onto Taylor. Go one block to 6th Avenue.

►Cross 6th to the corner of the Hilton Hotel.

►Turn right, cross Taylor, and pass the large steel sculpture rising from an oval stone pool, sometimes referred to as "The Bathtub."

►Cross Yamhill to your starting point at Pioneer Courthouse Square.

walk 3

South Park Blocks

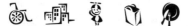

General location: The South Park Blocks are in downtown Portland, just west of Interstate 5.

Special attractions: Theaters, music, museums, indoor and outdoor art, varied architecture, and the Portland State University campus.

Difficulty rating: Easy, flat, entirely on paved sidewalk with curb cuts. The entire walk is wheelchair accessible.

Distance: 3.25 miles.

Estimated time: 1.5 hours.

Services: Restrooms are located inside the Tri-Met offices in Pioneer Courthouse Square and in all public buildings. Stores and restaurants are located throughout the area.

Restrictions: Tri-Met information center and the offices of Pioneer Courthouse Square Association are open Monday through Friday from 8 A.M. to 5 P.M. The restrooms are open every day from 8 A.M. to 7 P.M. Most public buildings have wheelchair accessible restrooms and are open weekdays from 9 A.M. to 5 P.M.

For more information: Contact the Pioneer Courthouse Square Association or the Portland Oregon Visitors Association.

Getting started: This walk begins at Pioneer Courthouse Square, between Broadway and 6th Avenues and Morrison and Yamhill Streets. From Interstate 5 northbound, take the exit to Interstate 405, then take the 6th Avenue exit and go south to Yamhill Street and Pioneer Courthouse Square. From U.S. Highway 26 eastbound, take the Market Street exit and follow the City Center signs to 10th Avenue. Turn left onto 10th, cross Taylor Street, and turn right onto Yamhill. Go three blocks.

There are three "Smart Park" parking garages in the immediate vicinity. One is on 10th between Morrison and Yamhill, one is at 3rd Avenue and Alder Street, and one is at 4th and Yamhill. These city garages offer the cheapest parking in town. Look for the red "Smart Park" signs.

Public transportation: Buses and MAX light-rail lines meet at Pioneer Courthouse Square. The Tri-Met information center and ticket office is below the coffee shop and is open Monday through Friday from 8 A.M. to 5 P.M. You can ride for free throughout downtown Portland. Contact Tri-Met for information about fares and schedules.

Overview: This walk begins at Pioneer Courthouse Square, center of downtown Portland and easily reached on foot from most downtown hotels. This square, scene of countless festivals and outdoor exhibits, is bordered by department stores, "vertical malls" of specialty shops within reconstructed buildings, excellent restaurants, and one-of-a-kind boutiques. The

South Park Blocks

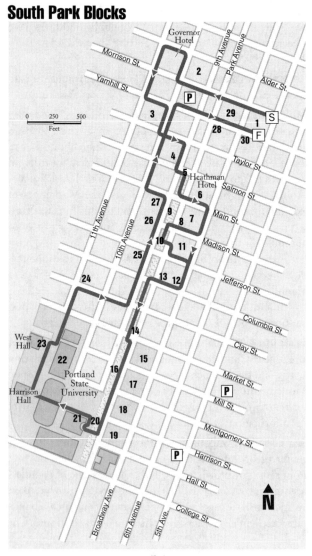

Points of Interest

walk continues through 12 tree-shaded park blocks, passing the newly restored Multnomah County Library, the Oregon History Center, the Center for the Performing Arts, the Portland Art Museum, and the campus of Portland State University.

The walk

►Start this walk at the Morrison Street and 6th Avenue corner of Pioneer Courthouse Square.

►Head west on Morrison. Notice the bronze drinking fountain with its four separate bubbling spouts of water. This is one of Portland's famous "Benson bubblers." Simon Benson, an early lumber baron and teetotaler, was disturbed to find his workers imbibing liquor during the day. When they pointed out that bars were the only nearby source of drink, Benson asked local architect A. E. Doyle to design a drinking fountain. Benson donated 20 of these to the city, strategically locating them near city taverns. The city installed others, and there are now 49 in the downtown area.

➤Continue on Morrison Street toward Broadway. Tall columns edge Pioneer Courthouse Square. These are a modern counterpoint to the traditional Corinthian columns on the bank building across the street. Just before reaching Broadway, you will see pieces of broken column lying on the ground. One piece supports a well-used tile checkerboard. The fallen pieces let you inspect the column details. You can see the tiny pink insects in the corners of the capital next to the stylized roses.

➤Continue straight to 9th Avenue. Cross 9th to the parking garage at the corner of 10th and Yamhill.

The Galleria vertical mall is across Morrison Street. Built in 1916 as a large department store, this structure was remodeled in 1976. Many interesting shops and restaurants are located around the original light well in the center of the building. What appears to be a transit shelter full of people outside the Galleria is actually another sample of Portland's outdoor art.

➤Continue to the center of this block, turn around, and look up at the parking garage overhang. Keith Jellum's *Electronic Poet* continually flashes "poems" of various words and phrases.

➤Proceed to 10th Avenue.

➤Cross 10th and then Morrison.

➤Proceed to the southwest corner of 10th Avenue and Alder Street. The Governor Hotel, built in 1909 and originally known as the Seward Hotel, displays more examples of terra-cotta ornamentation. Much of the original woodwork within the building remains intact.

➤Turn left onto Alder and walk to 11th Avenue.

➤Turn left onto 11th and go two blocks south to Yamhill Street.

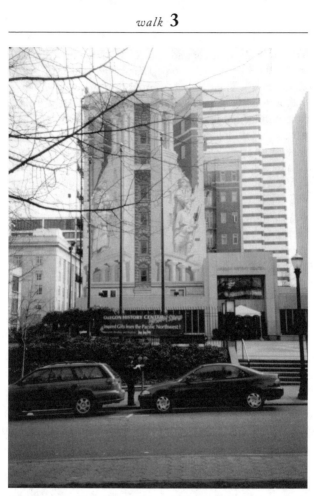

Oregon History Center.

➤Cross Yamhill Street and turn left. Proceed to 10th. The venerable Multnomah County Library fills the entire block on your right. The names of various topics and subject disciplines found inside the library are inscribed at the top of the building. These include fine arts, engineering, science, history, and philology, among others. Benches named after classic authors provide pleasant places to rest and read along the sidewalks around the library. These benches are one of architect Doyle's inspired solutions to Portland's sloping building lots.

➤Turn right onto 10th and continue past the entrance to the library.

of interest

Multnomah County Library

This timeless, classically designed building may be one of architect A. E. Doyle's most famous structures. It was completely renovated in 1997. Doyle's grandson, George McMath, was one of the architects who worked on this renovation. The interior walls were rebuilt completely. Most of the original decorations, columns, and wainscoting were retained.

The "Garden of Knowledge" theme came from the names of thinkers and authors inscribed on the exterior of the library and from the surrounding tall trees. It is reflected in the overhead garland adorning the lobby foyer, leaves etched into the steps of the grand staircase, and a wreath encircling the second-floor lighting fixture. The Beverly Cleary Children's Room has a delightful bronze tree in its center, with all sorts of sculpted natural-history objects hidden in the trunk. A sculpture of the artist's dog is at the base of the tree.■

➤Proceed to Taylor Street. Cross.

➤Turn left onto Taylor and cross 10th.

➤Continue to 9th Avenue. Look across Taylor to see the names and busts of musicians in the ornamentation on the Guild Theater.

➤Turn right. Go to Salmon Street. You are near the B. Moloch/Heathman Bakery and Pub. Look up to see the golden salmon leaping through the corner of the building. Directly across the street is a red-brick building with more terra-cotta ornamentation. This is the Arlington Club, once a private and exclusive club for Portland's influential men.

➤Cross Salmon and 9th. Take the wide curb-cut to enter the South Park Blocks.

➤From here, you have a good view of the statuary found in the next three park blocks. Go to the first of these, a fountain with low drinking bowls for pets. *Rebecca at the Well* symbolizes welcome, since the biblical Rebecca was noted for her hospitality and kindness to strangers and animals. A sign gives some history about fountain donor Joseph Shemanski.

➤Continue straight on this central walkway to Main Street. The building across Park Avenue on your left is the Arlene Schnitzer Concert Hall, part of the Portland Center for the Performing Arts. Formerly the Portland, a 1929 vaudeville and movie theater, it is now home to the Oregon Symphony Orchestra.

➤Turn left and cross Park.

➤Continue straight ahead on Main for one block to Broadway. You are skirting the south side of the Schnitzer. At the corner of Broadway and Main is the original canopy and sign for the old Portland theater, and to the left of this is the Heathman Hotel.

of interest

The Park Blocks

In Portland's early days, these blocks made a fine boulevard for carriages and horse racing. They were planted with grass and lined with elms in the late 1800s and were spruced up again during the downtown redevelopment. They provide a pleasant walkway through the center of the city and are lined with benches that provide comfortable resting places. There is a sculpture or fountain to enjoy in every block.

The original Portland founders intended this to be part of a 25-block parkway. Daniel Lownsdale and his partners, William W. Chapman and Stephen Coffin, dedicated the blocks south of Stark Street to the city. Benjamin Stark offered to donate the blocks from Stark north to Ankeny Street, and John Couch dedicated seven more blocks from Ankeny to Hoyt.

Unfortunately, Stark backed out of his agreement, and Lownsdale didn't leave a will. His heirs reclaimed the blocks between Salmon and Ankeny and sold them for commercial use. All but one—the O'Bryant Park block—still remain in private hands. Presently the park boulevard is divided into two sections: the South Park Blocks and the North Park Blocks, north of Ankeny Street.

In February 1998, a developer offered to donate the money to purchase the block between Taylor and Yamhill if Portland would come up with a park plan by the year 2000. Until then, it will remain a parking lot.■

➤When you reach Broadway, turn right and cross Main Street. The New Theatre building on this corner is also part of the Portland Center for the Performing Arts. It contains both the Dolores Winningstad Theatre and the Intermediate Theatre and has its own resident theater companies. If the building is open, it is worth a visit inside. Adorning the lobby is a gold and aluminum mural entitled *Portland Town*, by Henk Pander. A dramatic fireplace and a light dome are in the rotunda.

Free guided tours of both performing-arts buildings are offered Wednesdays and Saturdays. Contact the Portland Oregon Visitors Association or the Portland Center for the Performing Arts for information.

➤Follow Broadway south for one block.

➤Turn right onto Madison toward the Park Blocks. As you walk along Madison, look across the street at the Sovereign Hotel. The Oregon Historical Society uses part of this apartment building. Its plain brick facade has a varied terra-cotta trim, and the balconies still have their original wrought-iron railings.

The dark limestone wall of the First Congregational Church is on your right. Modeled after Boston's Old South Church, it was built in 1890. Many Portland citizens disliked this Italian Gothic structure when it was first built, and the dark basalt and light limestone pattern inspired the irreverent nickname of "the Holy Checkerboard." Only one of the lacy red and white towers remains. This is the only downtown church with a bell still in use.

➤Continue straight across Park Avenue to the center walkway in the park block. Turn around and look back across Park to better observe the church's architecture. From here, you can see how well the lines of the modern New Theatre building blend with the patterns in the church walls.

Look to your left to see the back of the Abraham Lincoln statue in this park block. Sculptor George Waters cast it in Paris. It has been criticized as being much too melancholy, but the sculptor said this was how Lincoln looked during the Civil War. Take a look for yourself, and then return to this spot.

►Cross Madison Street and go to the Theodore Roosevelt statue. In the 1880s, Dr. Henry Waldo Coe began practicing medicine in North Dakota and became one of Roosevelt's hunting companions. Coe later moved his practice to Portland. He chose Alexander Phimister Proctor, a well-known sculptor, to create this statue of his old friend. The bronze tablet at the base contains a wonderful tribute to the president.

Look left across Park Avenue. This side of the Sovereign Hotel, now the Oregon History Center, looks so three-dimensional that you would swear it was carved from stone. Richard Haas created the eight-story *trompe l'oeil* murals that are on two sides of the Oregon History Center. The mural on the front side of the building shows members of the Lewis and Clark expedition. If you look closely, you can see Meriwether Lewis, the slave York, Sacajawea and her baby Jean Baptiste, and Lewis's dog Seaman. The dog is 7 feet tall, which gives you some idea of the size of the murals.

►Cross Park Avenue to the Oregon History Center, headquarters of the Oregon Historical Society. You can enter the "Washington Ellipse" courtyard by the steps or by the wheelchair ramp on your right. The large sculpture, *Flying Together*, is by Tom Hardy.

It could take half a day or more to explore the museum's interactive exhibits and informative displays. The building contains an extensive research library, and the Oregon Historical Society also sponsors a press that publishes many books and pamphlets on Oregon history. Note the information about exhibits, hours, and prices displayed outside, or contact the museum.

➤Come out of the courtyard and continue south on Park to Jefferson Street.

➤Turn to your left on Jefferson and go to Broadway. A second mural on this side of the building depicts Oregon's development. You can see Native Americans, fur traders, and emigrants on the Oregon Trail.

➤Turn left and go to the OHS Museum Store. It has an excellent selection of nonfiction and fiction about the Pacific Northwest, including children's books. All gifts are either made in the Pacific Northwest or depict the region.

➤Retrace your steps south, cross Jefferson, and continue straight to Columbia Street. You'll pass the First Christian Church parking lot and a small gabled office building. This is the Ladd Carriage House, which once belonged to the Ladd Mansion. The original mansion was across the street where the *Oregonian* newspaper building is now.

➤Turn right at Columbia and walk one block back to Park. On this northeast corner is the First Christian Church. This is the only Portland pioneer congregation that still worships in a building on its original site. The present building was constructed in 1919.

➤Cross Park to the center walkway.

➤Turn left and cross Columbia.

➤Continue through the center of the next two park blocks. Notice the paving art, *In the Shadow of the Elm*, just before Market Street. It seems to reflect the elm across Market Street behind the sign for Portland State University.

➤Cross Market. The next six park blocks are part of the university campus. The cross streets are now pedestrian walkways. This busy and diversified university was originally founded to educate veterans of World War II. It was located in Vanport, a wartime housing development to the north on the Columbia River. When a 1948 flood destroyed the entire community, the college was relocated to the old Lincoln High School, now Lincoln Hall. It is the first building on your left.

➤Continue south on the center walk of the next two blocks. Cross the Montgomery Street walkway. *Farewell to Orpheus*, the fountain in this block, was designed by former PSU art professor Frederic Littman. Smith Memorial Hall is on your left. Publicly funded works of indoor and outdoor art enhance nearly every building at PSU. One of these, a mural commemorating Vanport, is located in the second-floor stairwell of this building. There is also a small art gallery.

➤Continue south past Smith Memorial Hall. The next large building is Neuberger Hall. *Oregon Country*, Tom Hardy's bronze sculpture screen, covers all the ground-floor windows. Intertwined ships, sand dollars, crabs, and plants represent Oregon's natural history.

The Millar Library is directly across the park from Neuberger.

➤Turn right on the walkway, pass the limestone sculpture called *Holon*, and continue to the library's circular portico. The wheelchair ramp is at the south end.

If the library is open, enter the lobby to view two different ceramic works: a large, colorful, and dramatic raku sculpture and a traditional, clay, wall sculpture memorializing former librarian Jean Black. The lobby sculptures are also visible through the large windows.

➤Leave the library and turn north to the walkway on the north side of the library.

➤Turn left onto this Harrison Street walkway.

➤Continue straight ahead to the end of the walkway at Harrison Hall on 11th Avenue.

➤Turn right onto 11th and go north to Mill Street. You will see the Department of Environmental Quality (DEQ) Laboratory on the east side of 11th. West Hall is on the southwest corner of Mill and 11th. *Cobbletale*, an interesting art piece, rises from the sidewalk in front. It was created from old streetcar rails, cobblestones, chunks of concrete, and other pieces of old city streets.

➤Cross 11th, cross Mill, and continue north.

➤Go through the cement barricades at Market Street, which mark the exit from the PSU campus.

➤Stay on the east side of 11th until you reach Clay Street. Directly across Clay Street, on the corner in front of you, is the Old Church. This is a beautiful and interesting example of Carpenter Gothic. Early Oregon had more woodworkers than masons, so wood was often used to imitate stone. A group of Portland citizens saved this church building from destruction. It's now used as a site for weddings and as a public meeting place.

➤Turn right. Stay on the south side of Clay.

➤Cross 10th Avenue. On your right is the South Park Square apartment complex. Notice the trees etched into its brick wall.

➤When you reach 9th Avenue, turn left and cross Clay.

➤Continue one block to Columbia Street. Cross. If you are observant, you will spy a small sculpture called *From Within, Shalom* located in front of St. James Lutheran Church. This echoes the *Peace Chant* sculpture of three stone slabs across the street in the section of the park block known as the "Peace Garden." Continue to Jefferson Street.

➤Cross Jefferson and continue to the entrance of the Portland Art Museum. The statue of Theodore Roosevelt is on your right across 9th, and you also have more views of the

Oregon History Center and the First Congregational Church tower.

➤ Pass the museum and continue straight on 9th. The Portland Art Museum's north wing, a large Greek Revival building, was formerly the Masonic Temple.

Notice the heavy and ornate bronze doors. The Masons supposedly modeled their temple on biblical descriptions of the one built by King Solomon.

➤ Turn left onto Main Street and proceed to 10th.

of interest

Portland Art Museum

Architect Pietro Belluschi designed the Portland Art Museum, as well as the museum's interior lighting. Belluschi's Northwest-style homes and public buildings reflect this area much as Frank Lloyd Wright's style reflects the Midwest.

The museum has an outstanding collection of Northwest Coast Indian art, Asian galleries with the largest West Coast collection of Chinese furniture, and other collections of art spanning several centuries. This is often the stopping place for national and international touring exhibitions. There is a gift store.

The museum's Evan H. Robert Memorial Sculpture Garden is just beyond the north wall. Several large pieces of sculpture are installed among the plantings and tall trees. In the back of the garden and to the right is the Pacific College of Art and the Northwest Film Center. The College of Art offers continuing education and degree programs in the fine arts, while the Northwest Film Center encourages appreciation of the "moving-image arts." Both have exhibits. ■

➤Turn right onto 10th and cross Main.

➤Continue straight on 10th for three more blocks to Yamhill Street. The east side of the Multnomah County Library will be on your left across 10th.

➤Cross Yamhill and turn right.

➤Continue straight east for three blocks. As you pass Nordstrom, notice the aluminum leaves along the wall— another bit of the public art that makes Portland so pleasant for pedestrians.

➤Cross Broadway to Pioneer Courthouse Square. From here, look across Yamhill for a good view of the Jackson Tower. It has been lighting up the Portland skyline since its construction in 1912. Outlining the building are 1,800 light sockets, which were built into the original terra cotta. The large clocks in the tower were battery operated and chimed every 15 minutes when the building was originally constructed to house the *Oregon Journal*.

➤Return to your starting point in Pioneer Courthouse Square.

walk 4

Chinatown and the Pearl District

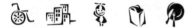

General location: Downtown Portland, west of Interstate 5.

Special attractions: Powell's Bookstore; the original Blitz-Weinhard Brewery; Chinatown restaurants and shops. The area is full of artists' studios; galleries; and fabric, antique, and home-decorating shops.

Difficulty rating: Easy, flat, entirely on paved sidewalks.

Distance: 3.5 miles.

Estimated time: 2 hours.

Services: Restrooms are located in the Tri-Met offices in Pioneer Courthouse Square and in all public buildings. Stores and restaurants are located throughout the area.

Restrictions: Tri-Met information center and the offices of Portland's Pioneer Courthouse Square Association are open Monday through Friday from 8 A.M. to 5 P.M.

For more information: Contact the Pioneer Courthouse Square Association or the Portland Oregon Visitors Association.

Getting started: This walk begins at Pioneer Courthouse Square, between Yamhill and Morrison Streets and Broadway and 6th Avenues. From Interstate 5 northbound, take the exit to Interstate 405, then take the 6th Avenue exit and go south to Yamhill Street and Pioneer Courthouse Square. From U.S. Highway 26 eastbound, take the Market Street exit and follow the City Center signs to 10th Avenue. Turn left onto 10th, cross Taylor Street, turn right on Yamhill, and go three blocks.

The "Smart Park" city parking garages provide the most inexpensive parking in Portland. There are three in the immediate vicinity. One is on 10th between Yamhill and Morrison Streets, with an entrance on 10th; one is at 3rd Avenue and Alder Street, with entrances on 3rd and 4th Avenues; and one is at 4th Avenue and Yamhill, with the entrance on 4th.

Public transportation: Buses and MAX light-rail lines meet at Pioneer Courthouse Square. The Tri-Met information station and ticket office—open Monday through Friday from 8 A.M. to 5 P.M.—is here, below the Starbucks coffee shop. You can ride free throughout downtown Portland. Contact Tri-Met for information about fares and schedules.

Overview: Portland's Pioneer Courthouse Square is the scene of countless festivals and outdoor exhibits. It is bordered by department stores, "vertical malls" of specialty shops within reconstructed buildings, excellent restaurants, and one-of-a-kind boutiques. The walk passes much of the sidewalk art

Chinatown and the Pearl District

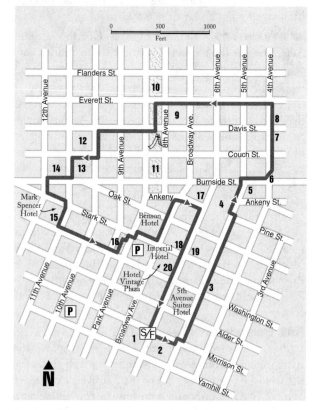

Points of Interest

 1 Pioneer Courthouse Square
 2 Pioneer Courthouse
 3 *Kvinneakt* sculpture
 4 U.S. Bancorp Tower
 5 *Car Wash* Fountain
 6 Chinatown Gateway
 7 Great China Seafood Restaurant
 8 House of Louie
 9 U.S. Customs Building
10 North Park Blocks

11 Children's Park
12 First Regiment Armory
13 Powell's Books
14 Blitz-Weinhard Brewery
15 Telegraph Building
16 O'Bryant Park
17 Lee Kelly Fountain
18 U.S. National Bank Building
19 Bank of California Building
20 Commonwealth Building

around the downtown transit malls. You will see Chinatown's unique shops and restaurants, as well as the art galleries, antique shops, and interior-decorating stores in the Pearl District.

The walk

➤This walk begins at Pioneer Courthouse Square.

➤Exit the square at the corner of Morrison Street and 6th Avenue, across from Pioneer Courthouse.

➤Cross 6th and go straight on Morrison to 5th Avenue. Pass the *Animals in Pools* sculptures by Georgia Gerber.

➤Cross Morrison and then 5th. Turn left onto 5th. A limestone sculpture, *Cat in Repose*, lounges gracefully on the sidewalk just before Alder Street.

➤Cross Alder and continue north to the center of the block. *Thor*, a riveted copper sculpture, can be seen across the street.

➤Continue to Washington Street and cross it. The sculpture *Kvinneakt* stands on this corner. This Norwegian "Nude Woman" gained fame when Bud Clark, who later became mayor of Portland, was photographed facing *Kvinneakt*, back to the camera and raincoat outstretched. The image was reproduced on a famous poster, "Expose Yourself to Art." An aluminum fountain sculpture, *Forms Found in Nature and in the Tools of Men*, is just beyond *Kvinneakt*.

➤Cross Stark and continue toward Oak Street. The Oregon Dental Services Building displays Manuel Izquierdo's sculpture *Unfolding Rhythms*.

➤Cross Oak and Pine Streets to a brick plaza. The U.S. Bancorp Tower, a Portland landmark, is across the street. Atwater's Restaurant, located on the top floor, offers marvelous views of the city.

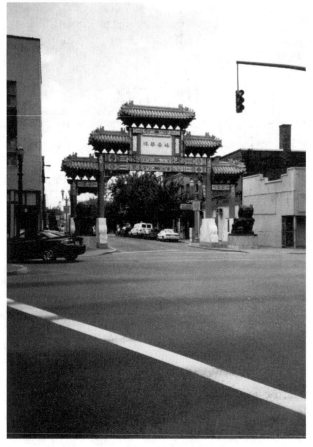

Chinatown Gateway.

➤Cross 5th to this "Big Pink" building. Turn right and continue to Burnside Street. Across 5th is a large, tubular, metal fountain nicknamed the "Car Wash." A wind gauge stops the water on windy days so that it will not be a traffic hazard.

➤Cross Burnside at the traffic signal.

➤Turn right to 4th Avenue. The Chinatown Gateway, dedicated in 1986, is an authentic reproduction of ancient Chinese gates. Plaques in both English and Chinese on the large marble pillars tell how and when the gate was given to Portland. On either side are large stone and porcelain lions. Look up to see the five roofs and find the 64 gold dragons.

➤Take the sidewalk on your right through the gate and walk into Chinatown. The red lampposts and signposts brighten the area. This area is especially beautiful in springtime when the cherry trees are blooming. There are two street signs on every signpost. The green one is in English, while the red one is in Chinese.

➤Continue for two blocks to Davis Street. At the corner of Davis and 4th is the Great China Seafood Restaurant. The House of Louie is across the street. Both are decorated with interesting Chinese motifs.

➤Cross Davis and continue along the west side of the House of Louie. Notice the little red roof on the telephone booth.

➤Continue north to Everett Street.

➤Turn left and cross 4th at the traffic signal.

➤Continue on Everett, crossing 5th.

➤Cross 6th Avenue. Continue straight past the Sally McCracken Building—another terra-cotta structure.

➤Cross Broadway. Walk past the brown U.S. Customs Building to 8th Avenue.

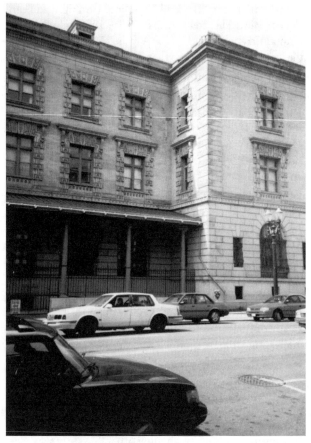

U.S. Customs Building.

of interest

The Pearl District

This area became a railroad warehouse district—once known as the "Northwest Triangle"—after Union Station was built in the 1890s. After World War II, most goods began moving by truck and the freight warehouses relocated to industrial parks by the highways.

The area slowly decayed until the 1980s, when artists—lured by cheap rent—began moving into the empty warehouses. Soon these were filled with loft housing and artists' studios, much like SoHo in New York. Art galleries soon followed. It was a gallery owner who renamed the district, observing that "much of the neighborhood's beauty is hidden behind crusty facades, like pearls in oysters."

Antique shops and furniture stores also relocated into empty ground-floor spaces, as did clothing stores, brewpubs, and small restaurants. New upscale lofts and townhomes are still being built in this now popular Pearl District. Even with the additional population, the district has kept its neighborhood ambiance. Many Portlanders visit on "First Thursday" each month, when the art galleries and other establishments on both sides of Burnside downtown stay open for the occasion.■

➤Cross 8th into the North Park Blocks and go to the central walkway. These blocks originally were intended to connect with the South Park Blocks. The lovely old elms arching overhead are among the few that survived an epidemic of Dutch elm disease.

➤Turn left and go south through the center of the block to Davis. Cross Davis at the crosswalk. A wonderful and well-used play area for children is located in the block between

Davis and Couch Streets. Originally, boys and girls were segregated in separate playgrounds; supervisors made sure members of each gender stayed where they belonged.

➤Turn right and cross Park Avenue.

➤Continue for two and a half blocks to 10th Avenue. Stop at 10th and look across at the building that resembles a white castle in a chess game. This is the First Regiment Armory.

➤Turn left onto 10th. Cross Couch Street. Turn right and cross 10th. You are walking along the back of Powell's Books, a well-known bookstore that covers a full city block. The store has more than half a million new and used books in its 43,000 square feet, as well as a large stock of magazines, newspapers, greeting cards, calendars, and book-related merchandise. There is a small coffee shop where you may snack as you read, and the store frequently hosts lectures, readings, and other events. The main entrance is on Burnside.

➤Turn left onto 11th Avenue. Pass the side entrance to Powell's. If you want to investigate, pick up one of the bookstore maps available inside. Books on different subjects are arranged in rooms of different colors.

➤Continue to Burnside Street. Turn right and cross 11th. In the middle of this block is the main entrance to the Blitz-Weinhard Brewery, the oldest in Portland. A sign outside the entrance marks a time capsule, placed here on the centennial of the brewery's founding by Henry Weinhard.

This young German brewmaster began brewing beer in Fort Vancouver in 1856. He moved to this location in the 1860s. The brewery, with its huge blue tanks, now covers several blocks. Thirty-minute family tours are available on weekday afternoons and include a stop in the hospitality room for alcoholic or nonalcoholic refreshment.

➤Continue to 12th Avenue and turn left. Cross Burnside at the traffic signal.

➤Go straight ahead one block to Stark Street.

➤Turn left on Stark. Continue east for one block, and then turn right on 11th. Pass the Mark Spencer Hotel and the red-brick and terra-cotta Telegraph Building with the corner clock tower.

➤Turn left at Washington Street.

➤Cross 11th Avenue. Continue for two blocks to 9th Avenue, passing by the Pittock Block Building.

➤Cross 9th into O'Bryant Park. This reclaimed South Park Block is named for Portland's first mayor, Hugh Donaldson O'Bryant. A large parking garage is below ground level.

➤Turn left and cross the plaza to see the rose-shaped fountain. This was donated by one of the Rosarians, a group of civic leaders who sponsor the annual Rose Parade.

➤Turn right to Park Avenue and cross.

➤Turn left and cross Stark Street.

➤Turn right and walk one block to Broadway.

➤Turn left onto Broadway. You are walking past the 1913 Benson Hotel, named for lumber baron Simon Benson. Architect A. E. Doyle copied the French Renaissance style of Chicago's Blackstone Hotel. Unusual bulls-eye dormer windows are under the mansard roof.

The Benson's lobby maintains its original grandeur. The original crystal chandeliers, walnut paneling, and marble floors give it a feel of Old England. A statue of a British Beefeater presides over small tables that look ready for high tea. Comfortable club chairs in a corner by a fireplace encourage sitting, chatting, and reading.

➤Cross Oak and go one block to Pine. Turn right and cross Broadway.

➤Continue to 6th Avenue. Sheets of water cascade over Lee Kelly's rust-colored steel fountain on the corner of 6th and Pine.

➤Turn right on 6th and go back to Oak. "Big Pink," otherwise known as the U.S. Bancorp Tower, is on the opposite side of the street.

➤Cross Oak and continue to Stark. The neoclassical U.S. National Bank Building on your right was built in 1917. The dramatic relief panels on its bronze doors were designed by Avard Fairbanks. The 1925 Bank of California Building across 6th is an example of the Italian Renaissance style.

➤Cross Stark. Pietro Belluschi designed the Commonwealth Building on your right, one of the first glass "curtain wall" skyscrapers. A small granite fountain with bubbling streams stands in front of this building.

➤Continue on 6th. Cross Washington and then Alder Streets. Pass by a geometric steel sculpture, *Talus #2*, which represents a legendary defender of Crete.

➤Cross Morrison. You are back at Pioneer Courthouse Square.

walk 5

Uptown and Nob Hill

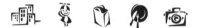

General location: The northwest section of downtown Portland.

Special attractions: City views, Victorian mansions, unique small restaurants, and trendy shops.

Difficulty rating: Moderate, with a few steep uphill sections.

Distance: 4 miles.

Estimated time: 2.5 hours.

Services: Restaurants, restrooms, and water.

Restrictions: This walk is not suitable for wheelchairs. Narrow sidewalks, few curb cuts, and uphill sections also make it difficult for strollers.

For more information: Contact the Portland Oregon Visitors Association.

Uptown and Nob Hill

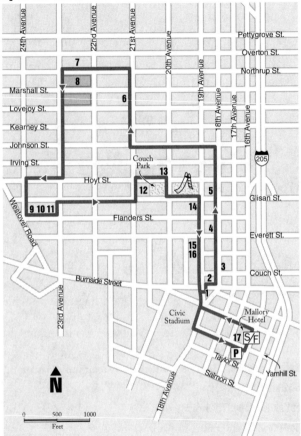

Points of Interest

1 Firemen's Memorial
2 McDonald's Restaurant
3 Cathedral of Saint Mary of
   the Immaculate Conception
4 First Church of Christ Scientist
5 Landenberger House
6 Cathedral of Saint Mark
7 Statue of Saint Francis and Friends
8 Good Samaritan Hospital
9 Bates-Sellers House
10 Charles Adams House
11 Trevitt-Nunn House
12 Metropolitan Learning Center
13 William Temple House
14 Temple Beth Israel
15 Trinity Cathedral
16 Cathedral Courtyard Garden
17 Lafayette Apartment Building

Getting started: The walk starts at the Mallory Hotel, 729 SW 15th Avenue. To reach the hotel from Interstate 5 north-bound, take the exit to Interstate 405 and then take the Salmon Street exit. From I-5 southbound, take exit 302B to I-405, then the Couch-Burnside exit. The hotel parking garage is on 15th Avenue, the south side of Yamhill Street. You can park there for a fee—or for free if you are staying or eating at the hotel. Metered parking is available on the street.

Public transportation: The MAX light-rail line stops at the Civic Stadium station on 18th Street between Yamhill and Morrison.

Overview: The Mallory Hotel is in the area once known as "Uptown." The "Northwest" district across Burnside was called "Nob Hill" by a grocer who wanted to associate this neighborhood with the well-known San Francisco district. It was a fashionable area for Portlanders whose desire for elegant mansions and large homes required bigger blocks and building lots. Now many of these surviving homes are filled with little shops and restaurants, giving two of the avenues the nicknames of "trendy-first" and "trendy-third."

The walk

➤Begin the walk at the Mallory Hotel's front entrance on 15th Avenue.

➤Turn left and walk half a block to Morrison.

➤Turn left on Morrison.

➤Continue for three blocks until you reach 18th Avenue.

➤Cross 18th to the wide sidewalk outside Civic Stadium. This 70-year-old arena plays host to local sports teams and is often used for special events.

➤At this corner, 18th and 19th Avenues join Morrison. Turn right and cross Morrison.

➤Take 19th Avenue, the left branch of the Y, and go down the hill to Burnside. The white marble structure on your right at Alder Street is the Firemen's Memorial, dedicated to Captain David Campbell and other firefighters who have died in the line of duty.

➤Cross Burnside at the traffic signal.

➤Turn right and go one block to 18th Avenue. Those with strollers and wheelchairs may prefer to go through the McDonald's parking lot since it is not as steep as the hill. A large mural of an Italian countryside is painted on the lot's back wall.

➤Turn left at 18th and go up the hill to Couch Street. Signs above the street names indicate that this is the Nob Hill Historic District.

➤The Roman Catholic Cathedral of Saint Mary of the Immaculate Conception is on the northeast corner of 18th and Couch. Built in 1925 and recently restored, this classic structure is graced with lovely bronze doors.

➤Continue north on 18th for two blocks to Everett Street. Cross Everett at the traffic signal. At this corner is the former First Church of Christ Scientist, built in 1909.

➤Continue north for two more blocks to Glisan Street. The name officially rhymes with "listen," but many pronounce it "Gleason." Just before you reach this street, you will pass the Elliston Apartments, built in 1889. The building is on the National Register of Historic Places. The house on the northwest corner directly in front of you is the 1896 Landenberger House.

of interest

Nob Hill

When this neighborhood began deteriorating after World War II, many of the old Victorian homes either were turned into apartment houses or totally neglected. Now this area is desirable once again, so many houses are being restored to their former glory. Some are single-family homes. Others house professional offices, some small shops, and restaurants. Many homes are listed on the National Register of Historic Places. The Queen Anne-style houses display a wide variety of windows, roof shapes, towers, turrets, and verandas—often in the same structure. The simpler Georgian and Colonial Revival styles of architecture are also prevalent. The district has more dwellers per block than any other city neighborhood, and residents are from all age, ethnic, and income groups.

The east-west streets in this area are in alphabetical order, making it easy to find a particular address. Most street corners have two-way or four-way stop signs, but a few are unmarked. Be careful when you cross the streets.■

➤Continue two more blocks to Irving Street. The old service station on the north side of Irving has interesting decorations set into the brick.

➤Cross Irving and continue to Johnson Street.

➤Turn left onto Johnson. The Ayer-Shea House at 1809 Johnson was built in 1892.

➤Proceed west three blocks to 21st Avenue. Your nose will inform you that you are entering a popular eating and shopping area. On pleasant days, outdoor chairs and tables line the sidewalks, inviting you to sit, eat, and watch passersby.

➤Cross 21st Avenue. Turn right, crossing Johnson Street, and keep going straight. The Anglican Church Cathedral of Saint Mark, a Romanesque church with a distinctive wheel window above the entrance, is on the corner of Marshall Street.

➤Continue to Northrup Street. Cross Northrup and turn left. Continue west for a block and a half, crossing 22nd Avenue. Across Northrup on your left are some of the buildings of Legacy Good Samaritan Hospital. The brick buildings on your right are part of the Linfield–Good Samaritan School of Nursing. Founded in 1895, this was the first nursing school in Oregon.

➤Turn right into the small courtyard between the two buildings and look for the statue of Saint Francis surrounded by five large birds. Then return to Northrup. Continue west to 23rd Avenue.

➤Turn left, cross Northrup, and proceed south on 23rd to Lovejoy Street. (If you need to use a restroom at this point, turn left and go to the 22nd Avenue entrance of Legacy Good Samaritan Hospital. Inside are wheelchair accessible restrooms and a drinking fountain. If you return to this area with a vehicle, you may park in the hospital parking garages on either side of Marshall between 21st and 22nd.)

➤Cross Lovejoy and continue straight along 23rd to Hoyt Street.

➤Turn right and cross 23rd. Go up the hill one block to 24th Avenue.

➤Turn left and go to Glisan Street. You will notice that at this point 24th Avenue merges with Westover Road.

The area to the south and west here originally was too steep for building lots, until a hydraulic company brought in earth-moving water flumes and sluiced unwanted earth down to the bottom of the hill. The dirt was used to fill in Guild Lake, once located near the Willamette River north of Vaughn Street. This former lake became the site for the 1905 Lewis and Clark Exposition. The company then terraced the hill and developed it as Westover Terraces, giving the streets aristocratic-sounding Virginia names.

➤Continue up the incline to Flanders Street.

➤Turn left onto Flanders. The next three old homes you pass are on the National Register of Historic Places. The Bates-Sellers House, with its large porches, is a good example of the Queen Anne mixture of styles. Note the Ionic capitals on the columns on the first story and the Corinthian capitals on the second-story columns. East of the Bates-Sellers House is the more classical Charles Adams House. The next one to the east, the Trevitt-Nunn House, displays a typical Colonial Revival symmetry.

➤Turn left at the corner of Flanders and 23rd Avenue.

➤Go one block north to Glisan. Turn right, crossing 23rd at the light, and continue on Glisan for two blocks to 21st Avenue.

➤Cross 21st at the traffic signal. Turn left, crossing Glisan and go one block to Hoyt.

➤Cross Hoyt and turn right. The large brick building on the south side of Hoyt is the Metropolitan Learning Center, located in what was once the Couch School. Children from all over Portland attend this public K-12 school. It has a unique project-based curriculum.

The turreted building at 2023 NW Hoyt is the William Temple House, now operated as a counseling center by the Episcopal Diocese of Oregon. This Richardsonian-style house was built in 1892 for Dr. F. William Mackenzie, one of the founders of the University of Oregon Medical School,

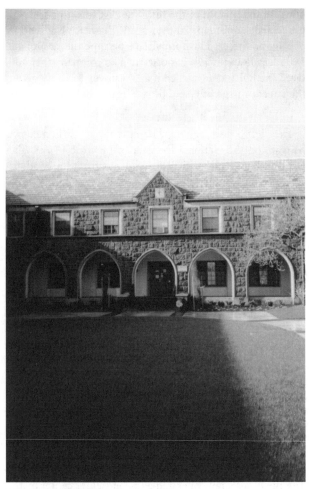

Trinity Cathedral Courtyard.

which was originally located nearby. The house is massively designed with a stone tower and windows recessed into rock masonry walls. There are many cast-iron embellishments, such as the sun decorating the stone chimney and the antlered stag—part of the Mackenzie family crest—peering down from an upper window. The front entry is around the corner on 20th Avenue. Scotch thistles are carved in the woodwork here, and there is a sign providing information about the Mackenzie family.

➤Turn right onto 20th, cross Hoyt, and enter Couch Park at the first walkway. Take the walkway south to Glisan. This park has drinking fountains, restrooms, benches under shade trees, and grassy mounds. David Kotter's tubular steel sculpture looks almost like a playground structure. Temple Beth Israel is across the street.

➤Turn left onto Glisan and walk along the edge of Couch Park to 19th Avenue.

➤Cross Glisan at the light. A Carpenter Gothic-style house is on the other side of 19th. You begin to see the towers of Trinity Cathedral as you continue up the slight hill.

➤Continue to Everett Street. Cross. On your right is the Trinity Cathedral of the Episcopal Diocese of Oregon. The cathedral's Rosales organ, described as "bright thundering, majestic," has 4,194 pipes and is considered one of the premier organs in the United States. Music lovers visit the cathedral to admire the organ; needleworkers admire the needlepoint kneelers. Designed and made by parishioners, each depicts a different Oregon flower.

➤Continue walking straight ahead. Go past the cathedral gardens, then down the modest hill to Burnside Street.

➤Cross Burnside at the traffic signal and continue up the other side to Civic Stadium at Morrison Street.

➤Cross Morrison and pass the stadium. Stop at the first traffic signal. Turn left and cross 18th. You are on Yamhill Street.

➤Continue along the little plaza on the south side of the MAX light-rail loading area until you reach 16th Avenue.

➤Cross 16th. The building at this southeast corner was once the home of Portland's Civic Theater. Across Yamhill is the Lafayette Apartment Building, trimmed with bas reliefs that look like Wedgwood pottery.

➤Continue east on Yamhill for one more block. Turn left, cross Yamhill, and you are at your original starting point at the Mallory Hotel.

walk 6

Circling Downtown

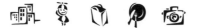

General location: Downtown Portland, west of Interstate 5.

Special attractions: Historic buildings, museums, parks, interesting shops and restaurants, and the Willamette River waterfront.

Difficulty rating: Entirely on paved sidewalks, moderately easy, some uphill slopes.

Distance: 6.5 miles.

Estimated time: 4 hours.

Services: Restaurants, restrooms, tourist information center.

Restrictions: Days and hours vary at the museums. The Portland Oregon Visitors Association Center is open six days a week, but hours vary. When the center is closed, maps and local information are available in an outside box.

Circling Downtown

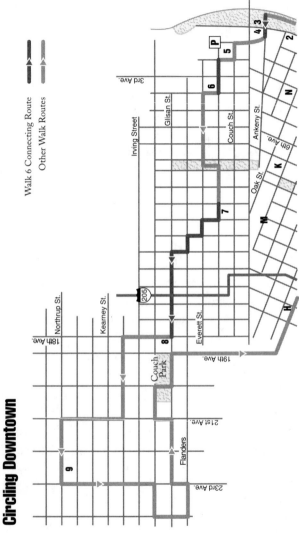

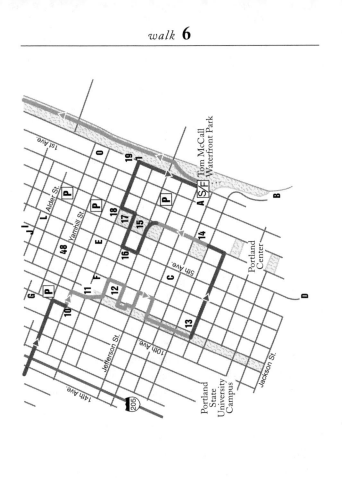

Hotels

A Marriott Hotel
B RiverPlace Hotel
C Days Inn
D DoubleTree Portland
E Hilton Hotel
F Heathman Hotel
G Governor Hotel
H Mallory Hotel
I Imperial Hotel
J Hotel Vintage Plaza
K Benson Hotel
L 5th Avenue Suites Hotel
M Mark Spencer Hotel
N Embassy Suites
O The Riverside

Points of Interest

1 Salmon Street Springs Fountain
2 Oregon Maritime Museum
3 Waterfront Park Story Garden
4 Ankeny Park
5 Fleischner-Mayer Building
6 House of Louie
7 First Regiment Armory
8 Landenberger House
9 Good Samaritan Hospital
10 Multnomah County Library
11 Rebecca at the Well
12 New Theatre Building
13 Lincon Hall
14 Civic Auditorium
15 Terry Schrunk Plaza
16 Portland Building
17 Chapman Square
18 Lownsdale Square
19 Portland Oregon Visitors Association

For more information: Contact the Portland Oregon Visitors Association.

Getting started: The walk begins at the Marriott Hotel between Clay and Columbia Streets at 1401 SW Naito Parkway. (Naito Parkway was formerly named Front Street, which is the name still shown on older maps.) From Interstate 5 northbound, take Exit 299B to Interstate 405, then Exit 1A to Naito Parkway. From I-5 southbound, take Exit 300B for City Center to the Morrison Bridge, then go south on Naito Parkway to the Marriott Hotel.

The "Smart Park" city parking garages provide the most inexpensive parking in Portland. A Smart Park is near the Marriott at 1st Avenue and Jefferson Street. Enter from Jefferson.

Public transportation: The Marriott Hotel is located within the downtown area, where you can ride city buses for free. Contact Tri-Met for information about fares and schedules.

Overview: This walk circles the downtown area, beginning at Tom McCall Waterfront Park in front of the Marriott

Hotel. Most downtown hotels are within a block or two of some part of this walk. It incorporates sections of Walks 1 through 5 to create a longer tour.

You will walk past historic buildings in the rejuvenated neighborhoods of Old Town, Chinatown, the Pearl District, and Nob Hill. Many of these older buildings—both businesses and homes—have recently been renovated, restored, and occupied by tempting shops and restaurants. You will also travel through the cultural center around the South Park Blocks and Portland State University, as well as the urban renewal area of Portland Center.

The walk

➤To start this walk, leave the Marriott Hotel by the door on Naito Parkway. Follow these directions until you come to the brick walkway just before the Waterfront Park Story Garden.

Leg 1

➤Cross Naito Parkway at the light. Continue straight ahead to the promenade along the waterfront, continuing under the Hawthorne Bridge and past Salmon Street Springs.

➤Continue on the walkway alongside the Willamette River. The large green park is Tom McCall Waterfront Park, named for a former Oregon governor.

➤Continue straight ahead toward the Morrison Street Bridge. The docking site for the *Portland Spirit* is on your right.

➤Go under the Morrison Street Bridge. On your right is the docking site for the sternwheeler *Columbia Gorge*. It and *Portland Spirit* offer river cruises.

Look down at the pavement to read the markers locating early sites in Portland history. The first one you see is for the Lownsdale land claim. The next marker informs you of the Stephens family land claim across the river. Farther north is the site of the first wharf, built in 1846. Next comes a marker for "The Clearing, 1840," with a picture of the way the area looked when Portland was founded. The "Indian Camps, 1845" marker follows.

➤Continue straight ahead. Watch for the USS *Oregon* smokestack on your left. This memorial to Spanish-American War nurses is from a battleship used during that war. A bicentennial time capsule, to be opened in 2076, is enclosed within the memorial.

A navy barge, *The Russell*, and the steamer *Portland* are moored along the seawall. The *Portland* was transformed into the "Lauren Belle" for the 1994 movie *Maverick*. You can buy a ticket to visit both ships at the Oregon Maritime Museum in the Smith Block Building, which is on your left across Naito Parkway; the museum contains two floors of maritime-history exhibits, plus a research library and museum shop. It is open year-round. Contact the museum for information about fees and times.

➤Continue straight ahead toward the Burnside Bridge. Before the bridge is a little square where a walkway comes in from the left. Ahead of you on your right is the Sculpture Stage. A red-granite throne marks the Waterfront Park Story Garden just ahead.

This children's "imagineering park" is designed specifically to encourage story ideas. Illustrated paving blocks punctuate a walking maze.

➤Turn left onto the brick walkway in front of the Story Garden and cross Naito Parkway at the crosswalk. Go straight ahead into Ankeny Park. More detailed descriptions of the buildings you will pass can be found in Walk 1.

➤Go to the colonnade at the far end of the square to see the antique Skidmore Fountain on the other side. Walk to the fountain. This is 1st Avenue.

➤Continue north, past the Blagen Block Building, to Couch Street.

➤Turn left and cross 1st Avenue to the Norton House, once a hotel where President Ulysses S. Grant stayed briefly. Signs will inform you that you are now in the Couch (pronounced "kooch") District.

➤Cross Couch and proceed west to 2nd Avenue. You will pass the 1906 Fleischner-Mayer Building, one of the first buildings restored by the Naito brothers.

➤Stop at the corner of Couch and 2nd. Look diagonally across at Erickson's Saloon on the southwest corner. Loggers and sailors once frequented its 672-foot-long bar. Supposedly, many drunk unfortunates were shanghaied from here.

➤Turn right onto 2nd and go one block to Davis.

➤Turn left and cross 2nd. Go two blocks to 4th Avenue. Turn right and cross Davis. You should be at the corner of the House of Louie restaurant.

➤Continue along the west side of the House of Louie. Notice the little red roof on the telephone booth.

➤Continue north to Everett Street.

➤Turn left and cross 4th at the traffic signal.

➤Continue on Everett, crossing 5th.

➤Cross 6th Avenue. Continue straight past the Sally McCracken Building—another terra-cotta structure.

➤Cross Broadway. Walk past the brown U.S. Customs Building to 8th Avenue.

➤ Cross 8th into the North Park Blocks and go to the central walkway. These blocks originally were intended to connect with the South Park Blocks. The lovely old elms arching overhead are among the few that survived an epidemic of Dutch elm disease.

➤ Turn left and go south through the center of the block to Davis. Cross Davis at the crosswalk. A wonderful and well-used play area for children is located in the block between Davis and Couch Streets. Originally, boys and girls were segregated in separate playgrounds; supervisors made sure members of each gender stayed where they belonged.

➤ Turn right and cross Park Avenue.

➤ Continue for two and a half blocks to 10th Avenue. Stop at 10th and look across at the building that resembles a white castle in a chess game. This is the First Regiment Armory.

Leg 2

➤ Cross 10th Avenue. Continue to 11th, passing the side of the armory building.

➤ Turn right onto 11th. Proceed one block to Everett Street.

➤ Turn left, cross 11th, and go to 12th Avenue. You will pass shops and galleries.

➤ Turn right and go one block to Flanders Street. At Flanders, turn left and cross 12th carefully at the stop sign. The train tracks running down the center of the street are still used between midnight and 5 A.M.

➤ Turn right, cross Flanders, and continue to Glisan Street.

➤ Cross Glisan and turn left. Proceed to 15th Avenue.

➤ Use the push buttons to operate the walk light at 15th. Cross 15th and then cross over the freeway, staying on the north side of the street.

➤Cross 16th and continue to 18th Avenue. New paint on the old buildings indicates that you are now in the Nob Hill District. The domed roof up ahead belongs to Temple Beth Israel.

➤Cross 18th. The 1896 Carpenter Gothic-style Landenberger House is at this corner of Glisan and 18th.

➤Continue two blocks to Irving Street. The old service station on the north side of Irving has interesting decorations set into the brick.

➤Cross Irving and continue to Johnson Street.

➤Turn left. The Ayer-Shea House at 1809 Johnson was built in 1892.

➤Proceed west to 21st Avenue. Your nose informs you that you are entering a popular eating and shopping area. On pleasant days, outdoor chairs and tables along the sidewalks invite you to sit, eat, and watch passersby.

➤Cross 21st Avenue. Turn right, crossing Johnson Street and continue straight. The Anglican Church Cathedral of Saint Mark, a Romanesque church with a distinctive wheel window above the entrance, is on the corner of Marshall Street.

➤Continue to Northrup Street. Cross Northrup and turn left. Continue west for a block and a half, crossing 22nd Avenue. Across Northrup on your left are some of the buildings of the Legacy Good Samaritan Hospital. The brick buildings on your right are part of the Linfield–Good Samaritan School of Nursing. Founded in 1895, this was the first nursing school in Oregon.

➤Turn right into the small courtyard in between the two buildings and look for the statue of Saint Francis surrounded by five large birds. Then return to Northrup. Continue west to 23rd Avenue.

➤Turn left, cross Northrup, and proceed south on 23rd to Lovejoy Street.

Note: If you would like to use a restroom, turn left here and go to the 22nd Avenue entrance to Legacy Good Samaritan Hospital. Inside are wheelchair accessible restrooms, and a drinking fountain. You may use the hospital parking garages on either side of Marshall between 21st and 22nd.

➤Cross Lovejoy and continue straight along 23rd to Hoyt Street.

➤Turn right and cross 23rd. Go up the hill one block to 24th Avenue.

➤Turn left and go to Glisan Street.

Across the road you can see what was once the entrance to the former location of St. Vincent's Hospital. You will notice that at this point 24th Avenue has changed to Westover Road.

The area to the south and west here originally was too steep for building lots, until a hydraulic company brought in earth-moving water flumes and sluiced unwanted earth down to the bottom of the hill. The dirt was used to fill in Guild Lake, once located near the Willamette River north of Vaughn Street. This former lake became the site for the 1905 Lewis and Clark Exposition. The company then terraced the hill and developed it as Westover Terraces, giving the streets aristocratic-sounding Virginia names.

➤Continue up the incline to Flanders Street.

➤Turn left on Flanders. The next three old homes you will pass are on the National Register of Historic Places. The Bates-Sellers House, with its large porches, is a good example of the Queen Anne mixture of styles. Note the Ionic capitals on the columns on the first story, and the Corinthian capitals on the second-story columns. East of the Bates-Sellers House is the more classical Charles Adams House. The next one to the east, the Trevitt-Nunn House, displays a typical Colonial Revival symmetry.

➤Turn left at the corner of Flanders and 23rd Avenue.

➤Go one block north to Glisan. Turn right, crossing 23rd at the light, and continue on Glisan for two blocks to 21st Avenue.

➤Turn left, crossing Glisan. Cross 21st at the traffic signal and go one block to Hoyt.

➤Cross Hoyt and turn right. The large brick building on the south side of Hoyt is the Metropolitan Learning Center, located in what was once the Couch School. Children from all over Portland attend this public K-12 school. It has a unique project-based curriculum.

The turreted building at 2023 NW Hoyt is the William Temple House, now operated as a counseling center by the Episcopal Diocese of Oregon. This Richardsonian-style house was built in 1892 for Dr. F. William Mackenzie, one of the founders of the University of Oregon Medical School, which was originally located nearby. The house is massively designed with a stone tower and windows recessed into rock masonry walls. There are many cast-iron embellishments, such as the sun decorating the stone chimney and the antlered stag peering down from an upper window. The stag is part of the Mackenzie family crest. The front entry is around the corner on 20th Avenue. Scotch thistles are carved in the woodwork here, and there is a sign about the Mackenzie family.

➤Turn right on 20th, cross Hoyt, and enter Couch Park at the first walkway. Take the walkway south to Glisan. This park has drinking fountains, restrooms, benches under shade trees, and grassy mounds. David Kotter's tubular steel sculpture looks almost like a playground structure. Temple Beth Israel is across the street.

➤Turn left onto Glisan and walk along the edge of Couch Park to 19th Avenue.

➤Cross Glisan at the light. A Carpenter Gothic-style house is on the other side of 19th. You begin to see the towers of Trinity Cathedral as you continue up the slight hill.

➤Continue to Everett Street. Cross. On your right is the Trinity Cathedral of the Episcopal Diocese of Oregon. The cathedral's Rosales organ, described as "bright thundering, majestic," has 4,194 pipes and is considered one of the premier organs in the United States. Music lovers visit the cathedral to admire the organ; needleworkers admire the needlepoint kneelers. Designed and made by parishioners, each depicts a different Oregon flower.

➤Continue walking straight ahead. Go past the cathedral gardens, then down the modest hill to Burnside Street.

➤Cross Burnside at the traffic signal and continue up the other side to Civic Stadium at Morrison Street.

➤Cross Morrison and pass the stadium. Stop at the first traffic signal. Turn left and cross 18th. You are on Yamhill Street.

➤Continue along the little plaza on the south side of the MAX light-rail loading area until you reach 16th Avenue.

➤Cross 16th. The building at this southeast corner was once the home of Portland's Civic Theater. Across Yamhill is the Lafayette Apartment Building, trimmed with bas reliefs that look like Wedgwood pottery.

➤Continue east on Yamhill for one more block.

Leg 3

➤Instead of turning left onto 15th, proceed straight ahead on Yamhill to 14th Avenue.

➤Cross the freeway and then 13th Avenue.

➤Continue straight for three more blocks to 10th Avenue. Cross 10th.

➤Turn right and cross Yamhill to the Multnomah County Library. For more detailed descriptions of the library and other buildings you will pass, turn to Walk 3.

➤Proceed to Taylor Street and cross.

➤Turn left onto Taylor and cross 10th.

➤Continue to 9th Avenue. Look across Taylor to see the names and busts of musicians in the ornamentation of the Guild Theater.

➤Turn right. Go to Salmon Street. You should be near the B. Moloch/Heathman Bakery and Pub. Look up to see the golden salmon leaping through the corner of the building. Directly across the street is a red-brick building with more terra-cotta ornamentation. This is the Arlington Club, once a private and exclusive club for Portland's most influential men.

➤Cross Salmon and cross 9th. Take the wide curb-cut to the entrance into the South Park Blocks.

From here, you have a good view of the statuary found in the next three park blocks. Go to the first of these, a fountain with low drinking bowls for pets. *Rebecca at the Well* symbolizes welcome; the biblical Rebecca was noted for her hospitality and kindness to strangers and animals. A sign gives some information about fountain donor Joseph Shemanski.

➤Continue straight on this central walkway to Main Street. The building across Park Avenue on your left is the Arlene

Schnitzer Concert Hall, part of the Portland Center for the Performing Arts.

➤Turn left and cross Park.

➤Continue straight ahead on Main for one block to Broadway. You should be passing the south side of the concert hall. At the corner of Broadway and Main is the original canopy and sign for the old Portland theater. To the left of this is the Heathman Hotel.

➤When you reach Broadway, turn right and cross Main Street. The New Theatre building on this corner is also part of the Portland Center for the Performing Arts.

➤Turn right onto Broadway and walk one block.

➤Turn right onto Madison toward the Park Blocks. As you walk along Madison, look across the street at the Sovereign Hotel. The Oregon Historical Society uses part of this apartment building. Its plain brick facade has a varied terra-cotta trim, and the balconies still have their original wrought-iron railings. The dark limestone wall of the First Congregational Church is on your right.

➤Continue across Park Avenue to the center walkway in the park block. Turn around and look back across Park to get a better view of the church architecture. From here, you can see how well the lines of the modern New Theatre blend with the patterns in the church walls.

➤Cross Madison Street and go to the Theodore Roosevelt statue. Then look left across Park Avenue. This side of the Sovereign Hotel, now the Oregon History Center, looks so three-dimensional you would swear it was carved from stone.

➤Cross Park Avenue to the Oregon History Center, headquarters of the Oregon Historical Society. You can enter the "Washington Ellipse" courtyard by the steps or by the wheelchair ramp on your right. The large sculpture, *Flying Together*, is by Tom Hardy.

➤Leave the courtyard, turn left, and continue south on Park to Jefferson Street.

➤Turn to your left onto Jefferson and go to Broadway.

➤Turn left and go to the OHS Museum Store. It has an excellent selection of Pacific Northwest fiction and nonfiction, including children's books. All gifts are either made in the Northwest or depict some aspect of the Northwest.

➤Retrace your steps south, cross Jefferson, and continue straight to Columbia Street. You will pass the First Christian Church parking lot and a small gabled office building. This is the Ladd Carriage House, which once belonged to the Ladd Mansion. The original mansion was across the street where the *Oregonian* newspaper offices are now.

➤Turn right at Columbia and walk one block back to Park.

➤Cross Park to the center walkway.

➤Turn left and cross Columbia.

➤Continue through the center of the next two park blocks. Notice the paving art, *In the Shadow of the Elm*, just before Market Street. It seems to reflect the elm across Market Street behind the sign for Portland State University.

➤Cross Market Street. The next six park blocks are part of the university campus. The cross streets are now pedestrian walkways. This busy and diversified university was originally founded in another part of town to educate veterans of World War II. After that campus was destroyed by a flood in 1948, the campus was relocated to the old Lincoln High School. This is now Lincoln Hall, the first building on your left.

➤Pass Lincoln Hall and turn left at the walkway.

➤Go straight to Broadway, keeping on the left.

➤Cross Broadway. Watch for traffic coming from the left. You are now on Mill Street.

➤Cross 6th. Traffic comes from the right. Continue past St. Mary's Academy to 5th Avenue.

➤Cross 5th, watching carefully for traffic coming from the left. Continue to 4th Avenue. Across the street is the Church of Saint Michael the Archangel.

➤Cross 4th at the light. Mill again becomes a walkway.

➤Take this walkway to the T intersection with the yellow metal sculpture appropriately called *Awning*.

➤Turn left. Go down the steps to Market Street. Cross with the light. You are on 3rd Avenue.

➤Pass the Ira Keller Fountain. The Civic Auditorium is across the street.

➤Cross Clay. The KOIN Center is on your right. The bottom floors house the KOIN television station, cinemas, offices, and small shops. The upper floors are luxury apartments.

➤Cross Columbia and then Jefferson. Turn left into Terry Schrunk Plaza. You can see the Liberty Bell replica and City Hall on your left.

➤Walk to the right around the brick circle to Madison Street.

➤Turn left, cross 4th Avenue, and go one block to 5th Avenue. Cross.

➤Turn right to reach the Standard Insurance Plaza. Look for the outdoor escalators and ascend to the lobby on the second level. From here, you will have a spectacular view of the Portland Building and the statue *Portlandia*. You are almost on the same level as the statue.

➤When you are through enjoying the view, take the escalator back down to 5th. Continue north to Main Street.

➤Turn right and cross 5th.

➤Stay on Main, proceeding past the Portland Building. The Multnomah County Courthouse is on the other side of the street. Pass the Elk Fountain between Chapman and Lownsdale Squares and go to 3rd Avenue. Stop to look at the Mark O. Hatfield Federal Courthouse across the street on your left and the Justice Center on your right.

➤Turn left and cross Main Street. Turn right and cross 3rd.

➤Turn left past the courthouse and walk to the corner of Salmon Street. Turn right on Salmon.

➤Continue two blocks to 1st Avenue. Cross 1st to the World Trade Center buildings. Continue on the walkway between the two buildings to the front door of the Portland Oregon Visitors Association. Volunteers at the visitor center can provide maps and literature, answer questions, and point out interesting items in the Made in Oregon shop. The Portland Oregon Visitors Association is currently housed in this building, but it plans to move to Pioneer Courthouse Square in 1999.

➤Exit on Naito Parkway and turn right. Cross Main, Madison, Jefferson, and Columbia Streets to return to the Marriott Hotel.

walk 7

Audubon House and Bird Sanctuary

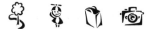

General location: Northwest Portland, west of Interstate 5.

Special attractions: Walk along Balch Creek through the Pittock Bird Sanctuary.

Difficulty rating: Moderately difficult. Dirt and gravel paths wind up and down slopes.

Distance: 1 mile.

Estimated time: 1 hour.

Services: Water, restrooms, nature store with an emphasis on birds and wildlife habitat.

Restrictions: Trails are open dawn to dusk. The Audubon House Interpretive Center and Nature Store are open from 10 A.M. to 6 P.M. daily, except on Sundays, when they close

Audubon House and Bird Sanctuary

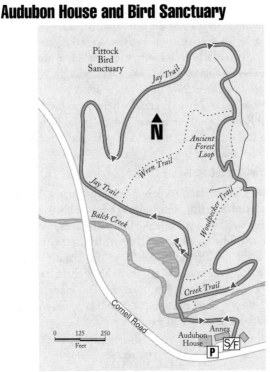

Special thanks to the Audubon Society for help with this map.

at 5 P.M. No dogs, smoking, bicycling, or littering permitted on the trail.

For more information: Contact the Portland Audubon Society and Nature Store.

Getting started: From Interstate 5 northbound, exit onto Interstate 405 northbound. Take this to the Everett Street exit. Proceed two blocks to Glisan Street. Turn left onto Glisan. Continue to NW 21st, go to Lovejoy Street, and turn left (west).

From Interstate 5 southbound, exit onto Interstate 405 southbound. Take this to the Glisan Street exit. At the first traffic light (on Glisan, a one-way street) continue straight ahead for two blocks to Everett, turn left, left again for two blocks, and left again onto Glisan. Continue to NW 21st, go to Lovejoy Street, and turn left (west).

Proceed past 25th Avenue where Lovejoy becomes Cornell Road. Continue west about 1.5 miles through two tunnels to Audubon House, 5151 NW Cornell, on the right side of the road.

Public transportation: None.

Overview: The Portland Audubon Society operates Audubon House, an interpretive center with exhibits of birds and wildlife. They also run a wildlife rehabilitation center specializing in birds. The excellent nature store features gifts, books, and aids for identifying the birds, wildlife, and plants you may see along the trail. A trail map shows three loop walks that begin at the store. The society offers many different birding events, nature classes, and guided tours, so call for information on times and dates.

The walk

➤Start your walk at the Portland Audubon House and Nature Store. Walk to the end of the covered walkway. The trail begins here.

➤Turn left onto the path at the end of the building and go down the stone steps to the sign that reads "Audubon Wildlife Sanctuary."

➤Go down more steps and over a small footbridge. You are descending to Balch Creek, a 3.5-mile, rain-fed stream.

➤Take the Nellie B. Stuart Footbridge over the creek. Birds singing overhead confirm this is a birder's paradise.

➤Follow the sign toward the pond. On your left just past the Creek Trail sign are some steps leading down to a rock with a bronze plaque. It explains that the little pond just ahead was named in honor of Samantha Jane Seaman, an Oregon Trail pioneer of 1852 who "cared for the birds for 75 years."

➤Pass these steps and take the lefthand path to Seaman Pond. Hawthorns and wildflowers border the path in season. Thick growth surrounds the still water. If you look carefully, you may spot some of the resident turtles and salamanders.

➤After investigating the pond, return to the gravel trail and continue left. Go past the entrance to the Woodpecker Trail, passing the tree with the picture of the pileated woodpecker.

➤Turn left onto the Jay Trail. This trail follows the north and east borders of the sanctuary. Boards cover the trail in places where the soil is soft. The vine maple here is easy to identify in the fall; it is one of the few Oregon native trees that turns red.

➤Continue up the path past the Wren Trail. Sword ferns and Oregon grape cover the bank on your right. You can hear traffic on Cornell Road as you go uphill from Balch Creek. The sound fades away as you continue around to the right.

Small licorice ferns grow on many trees. On your left is a large multitrunked clump of western redcedar. The branches on the outside surround a hollow center, now a bed for new plants.

➤Continue up the ridge past some small log markers. A glimpse of Cornell Road near the top makes you realize just how far you have climbed.

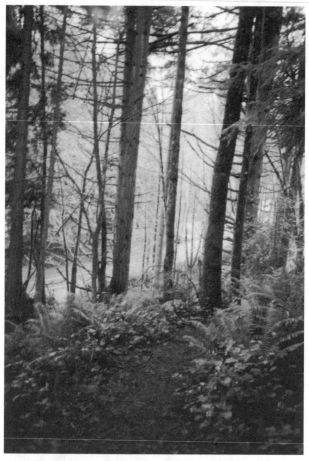

Looking down at Cornell Road.

➤Continue along the ridgetop on the narrow and twisting Jay Trail. Small rivulets trickle into Balch Creek. On both sides of the path are a number of stumps sprouting small trees and ferns.

You can see a storage shed above you on the left just before you start downhill. The trail goes around a fallen tree and then between pieces of another fallen log. Mossy fenceposts are on the other side of a little rivulet.

➤Cross the small footbridge to enter the old-growth area. These paths under tall firs seem small and almost hidden, making you feel like one of the early explorers. Decaying stumps and snags act as nurse logs for many new plants.

➤Continue to the spot where two trails join. The Wren Trail goes to your right. The next sign points to the "Ancient Forest Loop." Pass this sign. Ahead of you will be a small clearing with some fenced-off nurse logs. A stile takes you up and over one of these. Just beyond is a cedar tree with oblong holes drilled all the way to the top. This type of hole is made by pileated woodpeckers drilling for insects.

➤Retrace your steps to the sign marking the Ancient Forest Loop. Take this path to the left and go downhill to the T junction under towering old Douglas-firs. Look down to your right below the trail, where benches ring a small clearing.

➤Turn left at the T, taking the main trail to a fork. Take the trail to the left, crossing the bridge across a little stream.

➤Pass the entrance to the Woodpecker Trail and continue on the Creek Trail. You will see a sign pointing right to the Audubon House and the pond.

➤Take the path downhill, climbing over a dirt mound before turning left. You will cross a muddy area via wooden boards and pass an upended tree whose roots are packed with earth and stones.

113

➤Watch your step on the slope as you continue down to the little viewing deck. Audubon House is on top of the cliff on the other side of Balch Creek.

➤Continue on the path to a little bench with another view of Balch Creek.

➤Cross some duckboards onto a gravel path, turn left, and note the sign directing you back to Audubon House. Take the path and follow it back to your starting point.

walk **8**

Woods and Gardens Loop

General location: West of Interstate 5. This segment of the Wildwood Trail leads through a part of Forest Park in the West Hills above Portland.

Special attractions: A forestry museum, the Vietnam Veterans Memorial, the Hoyt Arboretum, the International Rose Test Gardens, the Japanese Gardens, and a garden of winter-blooming plants.

Difficulty rating: Difficult. The narrow, winding, dirt trail goes up and down wooded hills and may be muddy and slippery in spots after a rainstorm.

Distance: The Woods and Gardens Loop is a combination of four closed-loop walks totaling about 8 miles. It includes the Hoyt Arboretum Conifer Trail (Walk 10), the Vietnam Veterans Memorial (Walk 9), and the Japenese Gardens in

Woods and Gardens Loop

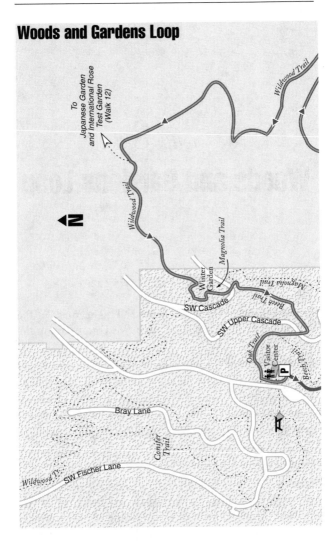

To Japanese Garden and International Rose Test Garden (Walk 12)

Wildwood Trail

N

Wildwood Trail

Magnolia Trail

Winter Garden

SW Cascade

Magnolia Trail

Beech Trail

SW Upper Cascade

Oak Trail

Visitor Center

P

Beech Trail

Bray Lane

Conifer Trail

Wildwood Tr.

SW Fischer Lane

116

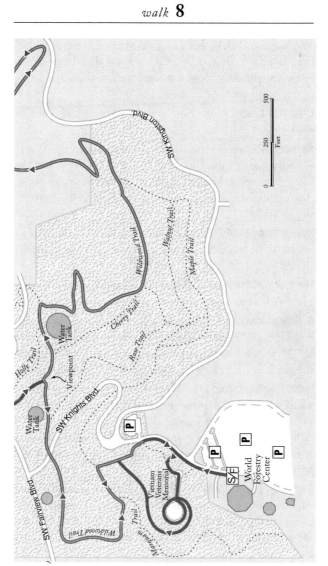

SW Kingston Blvd

Wildwood Trail

Walnut Trail

Maple Trail

Cherry Trail

Rose Trail

Holly Trail

Water Tank

Water Tank

Viewpoint

SW Knights Blvd.

SW Fairview Blvd

Wildwood Trail

Vietnam Veterans Memorial

Marquam Trail

Wildwood Trail

World Forestry Center

500

250

0

Feet

Special thanks to the Hoyt Arboretum for help with this map.

117

Washington Park (Walk 12). These three are connected by the 3.3-mile Wildwood Trail. You may walk all four closed loops together or choose the combination of loops that interests you most.

Estimated time: 6 hours for the entire Woods and Gardens Loop.

Services: Restrooms and water are available in the World Forestry Center, the Rose and Japanese Gardens, and the Hoyt Arboretum Visitor Center. Food can be found during the summer season in the kiosks at the Rose Gardens parking area.

Restrictions: No bicycles or motorized vehicles are permitted on these trails. Dogs must be leashed. No food is permitted inside the Japanese Gardens.

For more information: Contact the World Forestry Center, Hoyt Arboretum, or Portland Parks and Recreation.

Getting started: From Interstate 5 (northbound or southbound), take Interstate 405 to U.S. Highway 26 West. From US 26, take the exit marked "Zoo-Forestry Center." Follow the road to the parking lot for the zoo and forestry center.

Public transportation: The MAX light-rail (beginning in September 1998) and Tri-Met Bus 63 (Washington Park) stop at the World Forestry Center. Bus 63 also stops at the Hoyt Arboretum, the International Rose Test Gardens, and the Japanese Gardens. Contact Tri-Met for information about fares and schedules.

Overview: Forest Park, the country's largest, urban, forested park contains all six successional stages of a Western hemlock forest community. The park extends for 7.5 miles along the east flank of the Tualatin Hills, with an elevation of up to 1,100 feet above sea level.

Washington Park and the Hoyt Arboretum are among the seven individual parks included within the Forest Park boundaries. A wildlife corridor connects Forest Park with the coastal mountains, allowing the animal population to travel back and forth.

The Wildwood Trail stretches 28 miles from the park's southern boundary to its northern edge. Because it is fairly level, it is popular with joggers and runners. The surface is usually good, even during winter rains, and the trail provides a variety of views.

This walk begins at the World Forestry Center. It combines the walk for the Vietnam Veterans Memorial with the Hoyt Arboretum Conifer Trail and Washington Park walks.

The walk

➤The walk begins at the World Forestry Center Museum, which features permanent and changing exhibits on forests of the world, with special emphasis on those of the Pacific Northwest. All ages can enjoy the Talking Tree, the display of petrified wood, and the rain forest exhibit. There are also exhibits on woodworking, fly fishing, and firefighting. Visitors will gain a better understanding of what forests contribute to the world's well-being. The museum has a unique "Forest Store" with well-crafted wood and forest-related items.

➤After leaving the World Forestry Center follow the signs to the Vietnam Veterans Memorial. A path on your left goes up some steps and leads into the memorial. The ramped path for wheelchair access is a few yards beyond the steps.

➤Turn left on the concrete walkway lined with flower beds,

and go under a beautiful arched bridge. This takes you to the lovely Garden of Solace. Look up on the surrounding slopes to see the polished, black granite walls.

➤Follow the path on the left-hand side of the garden. This is the beginning of the spiral walk, which gently curves to your right. The path crosses the arched bridge, from where you can look down at the fountain and garden. Trees and shrubs from the dogwood and rose families border the circle path.

➤Continue on the path until you arrive at the first wall commemorating the years 1959 to 1965. Take time to read Terence O'Donnell's notes on each wall you pass—an excellent chronological reminder of recent American history.

This first wall represents the time during which the United States gradually intervened in the affairs of this former French colony, hoping to stop the spread of Communism. By 1965, the United States had 184,300 troops stationed in Vietnam.

➤Continue to the wall for 1966 to 1967, the years in which the United States became increasingly involved. Note the increase in the number of names of the dead.

➤Go to the 1968 to 1969 memorial.

During these years, North Vietnam began a major offensive, and President Lyndon Johnson decided not to seek reelection. His successor, President Richard Nixon, began withdrawing ground forces while increasing the air war. Names of Oregon casualties almost cover this wall.

➤Go to the wall for 1970 to 1971. Anti-war protests were evidence of a growing desire to withdraw from Vietnam, and the ground war was winding down.

➤Continue to 1972 to 1976.

North Vietnam occupied South Vietnam in 1975. The war was over. Only eleven names were added to the toll of Oregon dead during these years. In the previous ten years, more than 1.5 million Vietnamese and Americans died.

➤Proceed to the final wall. This memorial lists all those Oregonians who were still missing in action as of 1987. Stars mark the names of those whose remains have since been recovered.

➤After leaving this wall, walk down the path to an intersection with the Wildwood Trail. You have come about 1 mile. From this point the trail is not wheelchair accessible. You can return to your starting point by turning right toward the parking lot.

➤To continue on the next portion of the walk, turn left onto the Wildwood Trail. You will find many little benches along the Wildwood where you can sit and contemplate your surroundings.

➤Proceed to the junction with the Maple Trail. At the junction, turn left. You are now in a forest setting, a peaceful contrast to the memories of war.

➤Continue straight on the Wildwood Trail past its junction with the Marquam Trail. You have been going uphill on this section of the trail. Now the trail goes downhill as it turns to the right and continues through a grove of tall Douglas-fir trees. Glimpses of private homes on your left are reminders that this patch of wilderness is close to the city.

➤Continue on the Wildwood Trail as it turns right after the junction with the Hemlock Trail. A blue diamond-shaped mile marker is on the tree with the "Douglas-fir" sign. A sign on another fir tells you that you have come 0.25 mile from the trailhead. The trail continues uphill. You will come to SW Knights Boulevard.

➤Cross the road, watching carefully for traffic. On the other side is the sign for this National Recreation Trail.

In this area, different tree specimens are marked with "Flowering Tree Tour" signs. This is a self-guided tour. The guide is available at the Hoyt Arboretum Visitor Center.

➤You will see marker 17, just before the Wildwood crosses Rose Trail. Continue straight ahead on the Wildwood, passing the green water tank. Just beyond, on your left, you can see the red-orange bark of a madrone tree, and on your right is a little grove of Amur cork trees.

➤Continue up the hill past the sign for the Hoyt Arboretum Visitor Center. Stop at the viewpoint with the mountain-finder sign.

Neighborhood children call this "the top of the world," since there are great views on either side of the ridge. A sign on your left explains what you can see on a clear day. Directly in front of you are Mount Rainier, Mount St. Helens, and Mount Adams in Washington. Oregon's Mount Hood is hidden by the trees on your right. You can just glimpse Portland's famous Pittock Mansion between the trees.

➤Turn back from the viewpoint and continue. You will pass the Cherry Trail on your right, the blue half-mile marker, and the Holly Trail on your left.

➤Keep on the Wildwood Trail as it turns right around a water tower and goes downhill. Note the locustlike yellowwood with the "Flowering Tree Tour" label, and then Flowering Tree marker 9.

➤Stay on the Wildwood as it intersects once more with the Cherry Trail. You are still going downhill.

➤ At the junction with the Rose and Cherry Trails, by

marker 11, turn left, staying on the Wildwood Trail. A blue diamond-shaped sign marks the 0.75 mile point just beyond this junction.

➤Continue on the Wildwood Trail to the memorial bench for Nancy Jo Dawson at the intersection with the Walnut Trail. The ground and trees are covered with introduced English ivy. Though lovely and green, it allows nothing else to grow beneath it, and eventually it will kill the trees. Many volunteers are working hard to eradicate it, and there are different groups of "anti-ivy leagues."

➤Stay on the Wildwood Trail as it bends left, goes down-hill, and bends right. You'll see the blue 1-mile marker on a Douglas-fir.

➤Continue down to the bottom of the hill. There is a small grass clearing to the left of a gravel parking lot.

➤Follow the trail behind the posts edging the parking lot and go uphill into more Douglas-fir. You will pass a log used as a bench on the left side of the trail. Head downhill near a clump of birch trees.

➤The trail twists and turns uphill. You will pass the Douglas-fir with the 1.25-mile marker before dropping to SW Kingston Boulevard. There is a T junction at the bottom of this hill.

➤The Wildwood makes a sharp left turn away from SW Kingston Boulevard and takes a series of switchbacks uphill. Some large houses are on the slope above. As you pass the 1.5-mile marker, the trail looks as if it is climbing up to them. Instead, it bends back into the woods.

The trail flattens out as it follows the ridgetop. Look down the hill on your right to see the feathery maples and small pond in the Japanese Gardens. Tall holly trees soar up toward the trail.

➤Pass the 1.75-mile marker. There is a bench just before a sharp bend.

➤Continue around the turn. On the hill in front of you is a large, gray, boxy house propped up on stilts. Look for a low, green signpost on the left side of the trail. This is the junction with the trail to the Japanese Gardens. The Wildwood Trail continues straight ahead and back to the Hoyt Arboretum.

(*Author's note:* You have now walked nearly 2 miles. If you wish to visit the Japanese Gardens and the International Rose Test Gardens, follow the directions below. You can visit them and then catch Zoobus 63 back to your starting point. If you wish to follow the Wildwood Trail back to your starting point or take the Conifer Trail at the Hoyt Arboretum, follow the Wildwood Trail directions below.)

Japanese Gardens and International Rose Test Gardens Trail

➤From this green signpost on the Wildwood Trail, take the little trail downhill on your right. This goes to the Japanese Gardens. (See the map on page 161.)

➤The trail descends the hill on switchbacks. You will come to a place where the trail turns sharply left. A log railing provides a barrier on your right. Stop here and look down over the railing to get another view of the gardens. Note how every tree is pruned to perfection.

➤Keep on the trail to the bottom of the hill. Exit on the service road and turn right to the entrance to the Japanese Gardens. If you wish to follow a 1-mile loop through the Japanese Gardens, go directly to the entrance gate. There is an admission fee.

The Japanese Garden Society of Oregon began creating

these gardens in 1962. Designed by landscape architect Professor Takuma Tono of Tokyo Agricultural University, they are supposed to be the most beautiful and authentic landscape of this type outside Japan.

In less than a mile, you will walk through five different landscapes, each with its own distinct mood. The sound of water from fountains and waterfalls encourages slow strolling, quiet conversation, and frequent pauses. Each garden provides many changing views and is beautiful in every season of the year. Spring shows the pink and white blossoms of the cherry trees, the Japanese maples display every possible shade of red or orange in autumn, and the gardens' true serenity shows forth in the quiet greens of winter.

Many paths have uneven surfaces, making the gardens unsuited to those physically challenged. In the Natural Garden, stone steps take you up and down along waterscapes with small ponds, streams, and waterfalls. These can be slippery. Some of the pools are deep, and all are unprotected. Watch your children and your footing at all times as you navigate this particular area.

The Strolling Pond Garden has two sections. Crane sculptures and an authentic Moon Bridge are major features of the Upper Pond. The golden koi fish in the Lower Pond seem to enjoy people watching just as much as the people do. A zigzag wooden bridge takes you through iris beds and across the pond.

Weathered stones rise from sand raked carefully into wavelike patterns in the Sand and Stone Garden, while the sand in the Flat Garden resembles Japanese floor matting. Pleasure and happiness are symbolized by two mossy green plantings shaped like a saki bottle and a gourd bottle.

There is an outer Tea Garden where one waits for the tea ceremony, and an inner one surrounding the "Flower Heart" ceremonial tea house. A gift store by the entrance contains gifts, restrooms, and a drinking fountain.

If you wish to go directly to the International Rose Test Gardens, stay on the service road and continue down the hill. You will exit on Kingston Boulevard near the tennis courts, the gardens, and the stop for Bus 63, which will take you back to the World Forestry Center.

Wildwood Trail

➤From the green signpost on the Wildwood Trail (see the top of page 124), continue straight toward the boxy gray house. Stilts drilled deep into bedrock support the large houses on the ridge above.

➤The trail makes a sharp right turn. Pass the tree with the 2-mile marker. Continue up the hill. Near the top of the hill, you will reenter the Hoyt Arboretum.

➤Turn right by a drainage culvert and continue around the bend to where the Magnolia Trail intersects the Wildwood.

➤Turn left onto the Magnolia Trail and enter the Winter Garden whose plants bloom in winter.

➤Pass the bench given in memory of James Mitchell Taylor and inscribed with a quotation from poet e. e. cummings. A corkscrew hazel marks the junction of the trail and SW Cascade Road. A beautiful clump of white-barked Himalayan birch is on your left.

➤Cross the road and start up the hill on the Magnolia Trail. Almost immediately, you will come to the Beech Trail junction.

➤Turn left onto Beech Trail. Keep going straight past some magnolia trees. The trail turns right at an American beech tree and then crosses SW Upper Cascade Road.

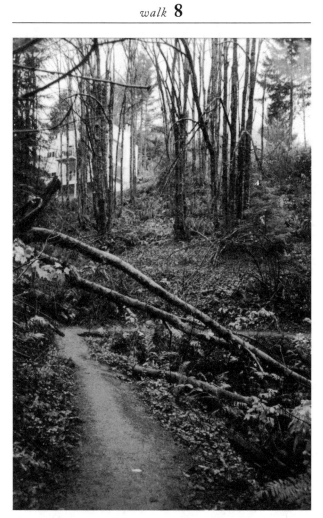

On Wildwood Trail, just past the turnoff to the Japanese Gardens.

➤Cross the road and take the wooden steps up the hill to where the trail meets the Oak Trail. Notice marker 3 for the Flowering Tree Tour. Information for this self-guided nature trail can be found at the Hoyt Arboretum Visitor Center.

➤Turn right onto Oak Trail, and then turn left. The visitor center should be on your left. Pass marker 1 of the Flowering Tree Tour.

➤Oak Trail ends at SW Fairview Boulevard. Turn left to the visitor center, where water, restrooms, and trail information can be found. You have walked 2.5 miles to this point.

➤If you wish to follow the 1-mile Conifer Trail, follow these directions. (See the map on page 142.) Otherwise, pick up the Wildwood Trail directions on page 130.

Conifer Trail

➤From the front door of the visitor center, cross Fairview Boulevard at the crosswalk and take the steps down to the picnic shelter. The conifer tour begins on the Spruce Trail, to the right of the shelter's drinking fountain.

➤Look for the marker 1 post. The salal bush, common west of the Cascades, has leathery leaves and pink flowers. Birds and small mammals eat the purple berries, which were also used as food by Native Americans.

➤The Spruce Trail goes to the left of this bush.

Notice the small identification signs placed on nearly all the trees. You will pass some Manchurian firs before you come to marker 2 at a Douglas-fir. The cones of this tree hang down from the branches, instead of standing upright, and botanists do not consider it to be a true fir. Common west of the Cascades, the Douglas-fir is one of the most preferred trees for lumber.

Look at one of the cones. Can you see the bracts sticking out from the scales? Jill Schatz's booklet, *Conifer Tour: A Self-Guided Nature Walk*, describes these as being like the tails of mice sheltering from an Oregon rain.

➤Cross SW Fischer Lane and continue down the path to your right, past the Himalayan spruce at marker 3.

➤The path goes left at marker 4. At marker 5, a bench given in memory of John C. Cahalan sits under a Sitka spruce. The Spruce Trail sign is across from the bench.

➤Go straight and then left through a grove of Norway spruce. Look for the bench. Take the path to your right, go down a hill, and come out on the south side of the "Wedding Meadow." Tables invite you to picnic here. It is a popular spot for weddings because all the flowering plants here have white blossoms.

➤A bench remembering "Sniffles" is on your right by the ponderosa pine at marker 8. Continue straight on the Spruce Trail, crossing the Yellow Pine Trail. A sign at marker 9 gives some facts about pines, as well as a brief note about a mythological Greek goddess who reportedly cared for these trees. The beads of pitch on pine trees are said to be her tears.

➤Pass marker 9 and continue to 10. Note the two strange-looking weeping sequoias that creep along the ground by upright ones.

➤The Spruce Trail meets the Wildwood Trail near marker 12. Turn left onto the Wildwood, a popular jogging trail.

➤Go downhill through the tall sequoias of a redwood forest. A bench at the bend to the left is dedicated to two beloved dogs. A sign begins, "Go to the first star. Turn right. Head straight on till morning." Past this bench is another junction where the Wildwood Trail goes downhill to the right.

➤At the junction of Wildwood and Redwood Trails, keep straight on Redwood Trail, going under a Port Orford cedar. Pass a bench by marker 17 and then a western redcedar. Ignore the path leading down to the creek at marker 19 and continue to the Cedar of Lebanon at marker 20.

➤You will cross another trail. Bear right to marker 22. A grassy uphill slope is on your left. Marker 24 identifies a Deodar cedar shortly before you reach SW Fischer Lane.

➤Cross SW Fischer Lane, watching carefully for traffic. Continue on the path on the other side. The memorial bench for John M. Bond is underneath a Japanese larch tree at marker 26.

➤The path goes uphill to your right through a variety of firs. You will pass a tall Noble fir, sometimes called an "Oregon Larch."

➤Go straight ahead past the junction with the Fir Trail. The picnic shelter is just ahead.

➤Turn right at the shelter and return across Fairview Boulevard to the visitor center.

Wildwood Trail

➤To return to your starting point at the World Forestry Center, continue past the visitor center to the large parking lot.

➤Turn left into the parking lot. Look for the service road going up the hill on your right.

➤Cross the lot to this service road. It is marked with signs reading "No Private Vehicles Beyond This Point" and "No Bicycles, Please."

➤Take this road up the hill until you rejoin Wildwood Trail.

The Wildwood Trail viewpoint will be on your left.

➤Turn right onto the Wildwood. Go past the reservoir and retrace your steps to the trailhead by the parking lot at the junction of SW Knights Boulevard and SW Kingston Boulevard.

➤Turn right onto the sidewalk.

➤Follow the sidewalk back to your starting point at the World Forestry Center.

walk 9

Vietnam Veterans Memorial and the World Forestry Center

General location: Northwest Portland, near the Washington Park Zoo.

Special attractions: A museum devoted to forests and forest products, a memorial to Oregon's Vietnam veterans, and a tour through part of the Hoyt Arboretum. The parking lot at the starting point also serves the Oregon Zoo, so you may want to add this to the tour.

Difficulty rating: Moderately easy. The tour through the Vietnam memorial is wheelchair accessible. The paved trail has an easy grade. The Wildwood Trail is narrow and dirt, not suitable for wheelchairs.

Distance: 2 miles.

Estimated time: 1 hour.

Services: Water and wheelchair-accessible restrooms are available at the World Forestry Center. There is a restaurant at the zoo. However, to eat there, you must first pay the zoo admission fee.

Restrictions: In respect for those who come to the memorial seeking solace, visitors are asked to limit active recreation to areas outside the Memorial Bowl. No sledding, off-trail skiing, or alcoholic beverages.

For more information: Contact the World Forestry Center or the Hoyt Arboretum.

Getting started: From Interstate 5 (northbound or southbound) take Interstate 405 to U.S. Highway 26 westbound. Then take the exit marked "Zoo-Forestry Center" and follow the road to the parking lot of the zoo/forestry center at the MAX light-rail station (opening September 1998).

Public transportation: Tri-Met Bus 63 (Washington Park) and the MAX light-rail train stop at the World Forestry Center. Contact Tri-Met for information about fares and schedules.

Overview: The World Forestry Center features permanent and changing exhibits on forests of the world, with special emphasis on those of the Pacific Northwest. All ages can enjoy the Talking Tree, the display of petrified wood, and the rain-forest exhibit. There are also exhibits of particular interest to woodworkers, fly fishers, and firefighters. Visitors will gain a better understanding of what forests contribute to the world's equilibrium. The museum has a unique "Forest Store" with well-crafted wood and forest-related items.

The Vietnam Veterans of Oregon Memorial was erected in 1989 as a tribute to those Oregonians who fought in that

Vietnam Veterans Memorial and the World Forestry Center

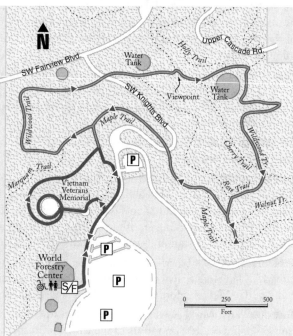

undeclared war. Often considered to be similar to the Vietnam Memorial in Washington, D.C., it is actually quite different in arrangement and mood. The walls are of the same polished black granite as the Washington memorial, and the names are engraved in the same fashion. The walls are carefully positioned on a path that spirals around the Garden of Solace and up the hillside like grooves on a giant snail shell.

Each short stretch of wall covers a particular period of the Vietnam War. The center part of each is a memorial to those Oregonians who died during these years. Comments on a stone on top of each wall tell about war events. The side panels tell what was going on in these soldiers' hometowns while they were away, giving poignant glimpses into daily events both "momentous and trivial, comic and tragic." Author and historian Terence O'Donnell wrote the brief episodes. The accounts bring history to life, and visitors born long after this war should find this an interesting view of the past.

The walk

➤Start at the World Forestry Center and follow the signs to the Vietnam Veterans of Oregon Memorial. A path on your left goes up some steps and leads into the memorial. The ramped path for wheelchair access is a few yards beyond the steps.

➤Turn left onto the concrete walkway lined with flower beds and go under a beautiful arched bridge. This takes you to the lovely Garden of Solace. Look up on the surrounding slopes to see the polished, black-granite walls.

➤Follow the path on the left-hand side of the garden. This is the beginning of a gently spiraling walkway. The path crosses the arched bridge, from which you can view the fountain and garden. Trees and shrubs from the dogwood and rose families border the circular path.

➤Continue on the path until you arrive at the first wall commemorating the years 1959 to 1965. Take time to read the notes on each wall as you pass—they are an excellent chronological reminder of recent American history.

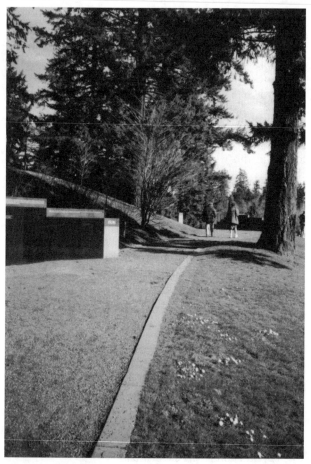

Walking to the MIA wall.

This first wall represents the time during which the United States gradually intervened in the affairs of this former French colony, hoping to stop the spread of Communism. By 1965, the United States had 184,300 troops stationed in Vietnam.

➤Continue to the wall for 1966 to 1967, the years in which the United States became increasingly involved. Note the increase in the number of names of the dead.

➤Go to the 1968 to 1969 memorial. During these years, North Vietnam began a major offensive, and President Lyndon Johnson decided not to seek reelection. His successor, President Richard Nixon, began withdrawing ground forces while increasing the air war. Names of Oregon casualties almost cover this wall.

➤Go to the wall for 1970 to 1971. Anti-war protests were evidence of a growing desire to withdraw from Vietnam, and the ground war was winding down.

➤Continue to 1972 to 1976. North Vietnam occupied South Vietnam in 1975. The war was over. Only eleven names were added to the toll of Oregon dead during these years. In the previous ten years, more than 1.5 million Vietnamese and Americans died.

➤Proceed to the final wall. This memorial lists all those Oregonians who were still missing in action as of 1987. Stars mark the names of those whose remains have since been recovered.

➤After leaving this wall, walk down the path to an intersection with the Wildwood Trail. You have come about 1 mile. From this point the trail is not wheelchair accessible. You can return to your starting point by turning right toward the parking lot.

➤To continue on the next portion of the walk, turn left onto the Wildwood Trail. You will find many little benches along Wildwood where you can sit and contemplate your surroundings.

➤Proceed to the junction with the Maple Trail. At the junction, turn left. You are now in a forest setting, a peaceful contrast to the memories of war.

➤Continue straight on Wildwood Trail past its junction with Marquam Trail. You have been going uphill on this section of the trail. Now the trail goes downhill as it turns to the right and continues through a grove of tall Douglas-fir trees. Glimpses of private homes on your left are reminders that this patch of wilderness is close to the city.

➤Continue on Wildwood Trail as it turns right after the junction with the Hemlock Trail. A blue diamond-shaped mile marker is on the tree with the "Douglas-fir" sign. A sign on another fir tells you that you have come 0.25 mile from the trailhead. The trail continues uphill. You will come to SW Knights Boulevard.

➤Cross the road, watching carefully for traffic. On the other side is the sign for this National Recreation Trail.

In this area, different tree specimens are marked with "Flowering Tree Tour" signs. This is a self-guided tour. The guide is available at the Hoyt Arboretum Visitor Center.

➤You will see marker 17, just before the Wildwood crosses the Rose Trail. Continue straight ahead on the Wildwood, passing the green water tank. Just beyond, on your left, you can see the red-orange bark of a madrone tree, and on your right is a little grove of Amur cork trees.

➤Continue up the hill past the sign for the Hoyt Arboretum Visitor Center. Stop at the viewpoint with the mountain-finder sign.

Neighborhood children call this "the top of the world," since there are great views on either side of the ridge. A sign on your left explains what you can see on a clear day. Directly in front of you are Mount Rainier, Mount St. Helens, and Mount Adams in Washington. Oregon's Mount Hood is hidden by the trees on your right. You can just glimpse Portland's famous Pittock Mansion between the trees.

➤Turn back from the viewpoint and continue. You will pass Cherry Trail on your right, the blue half-mile marker, and Holly Trail on your left.

➤Keep on the Wildwood Trail as it turns right around a water tower and goes downhill. Note the locustlike yellowwood with the "Flowering Tree Tour" label, and then Flowering Tree marker 9.

➤Stay on Wildwood as it intersects once more with Cherry Trail. You are still going downhill.

➤At the junction with the Rose and Cherry Trails, take the Rose Trail. Marker 11 identifies an American smoke tree.

➤Pass a bench marked with the initials P.M.W. The trail goes through more Douglas-fir trees.

➤Turn left at the junction with the Hawthorn Trail. Pass through a grove of hawthorn trees as you go downhill to the intersection with the Walnut Trail.

➤Turn right onto the narrow Walnut Trail. There is a lovely meadow up ahead. On your right is a Vulcan maple.

➤The Walnut Trail intersects the Maple Trail. Take the Maple to your right. Stands of birches and tall poplars edge the trail. Just beyond, you will come to some maples, followed by a green ash tree, some firs, and western redcedars.

➤The trail crosses SW Knights Boulevard. Continue straight ahead on the Maple Trail until it ends at a junction with the Wildwood Trail.

➤Turn left onto the Wildwood Trail and follow it downhill to the parking lot of the World Forestry Center. The sign at this trailhead, "Wild in the City," tells about the park's founding and shows the network of trails that wind through Forest Park.

➤Stay on the sidewalk and return to the forestry center.

walk 10
The Hoyt Arboretum
Conifer Trail

General location: Hoyt Arboretum is on the west side of Portland.

Special attractions: A sylvan retreat containing the world's largest collection of conifers.

Difficulty rating: Moderately easy dirt trail with one uphill section.

Distance: 1 mile.

Estimated time: 45 minutes.

Services: Water, picnic shelter, picnic tables, visitor center with exhibits, a horticultural library, and a small shop with tree-related gifts and books. A few snacks are also available. The wheelchair-accessible restrooms remain open until the park closes at 10 P.M.

141

The Hoyt Arboretum Conifer Trail

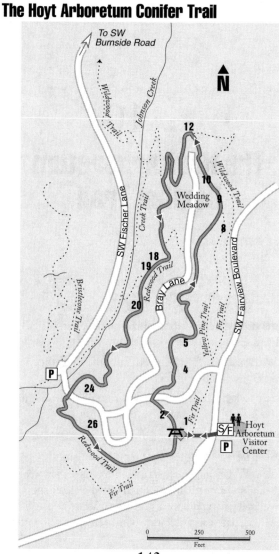

Restrictions: The center is staffed by volunteers and is generally open each day. Visitors are prohibited from picking any plants. No fires or alcoholic beverages are allowed in the park. Mountain bikes and motorized vehicles are prohibited on the trails.

For more information: Contact the Hoyt Arboretum.

Getting started: From downtown Portland, take U.S. Highway 26 westbound to the Zoo-Forestry Center exit. Follow the signs to the Hoyt Arboretum Visitor Center at 4000 SW Fairview Boulevard. You can also take Burnside Street west to the arboretum by following the entrance sign on the left about a mile west of NW 23rd. Keep following the signs to the arboretum. The main parking lot is on the south side of the visitor center.

Public transportation: Bus 63 (Washington Park) from downtown Portland stops at the Hoyt Arboretum Visitor Center. Contact Tri-Met for information about schedules and fares.

Overview: Stroll through the largest assortment of conifers in the world and see various species of redwood, spruce, fir, cedar, and pine. The Hoyt Arboretum features more than 800 labeled species of trees and shrubs spread out over 175 acres. There are 8 miles of trails within the arboretum itself, and some of these connect with other trails in Forest Park. Guided weekend nature walks are offered from April through October.

This was once the original site of the Multnomah County poor farm. Now it is a scientific garden and tree museum, as well as a public park. When the arboretum was established in 1931, its founders saved as many of the natural trees as possible. As plants from every continent of the world except Antarctica were added, they were carefully interspersed among the natives. Ten different trails exhibit different tree species.

143

The Conifer Trail combines the Spruce and Redwood Trails into one walk among the evergreens of the Northwest. Open pine and spruce forests contrast with the denser growth of the coastal redwoods. The visitor center sells an annotated nature-trail booklet by Jill Schatz, *Conifer Tour: A Self-Guided Nature Walk*, which has excellent explanations for every marker on the trail, as well as botanical drawings.

The walk

➤From the front door of the visitor center, cross Fairview Boulevard at the crosswalk and take the steps down to the picnic shelter. The conifer tour begins on the Spruce Trail, to the right of the shelter's drinking fountain.

➤Look for the marker 1 post. The salal bush, common west of the Cascades, has leathery leaves and pink flowers. Birds and small mammals eat the purple berries, which were also used as food by Native Americans.

➤The Spruce Trail goes to the left of this bush.

Notice the small identification signs placed on nearly all the trees. You will pass some Manchurian firs before you come to marker 2 at a Douglas-fir. The cones of this tree hang down from the branches, instead of standing upright, and botanists do not consider it to be a true fir. Common west of the Cascades, the Douglas-fir is one of the most preferred trees for lumber.

Look at one of the cones. Can you see the bracts sticking out from the scales? Schatz's booklet describes these as being like the tails of mice sheltering from an Oregon rain.

➤Cross SW Fischer Lane and continue down the path to your right, past the Himalayan spruce at marker 3.

➤The path goes left at marker 4. At marker 5, a bench given in memory of John C. Cahalan sits under a Sitka spruce. The Spruce Trail sign is across from the bench.

➤Go straight and then left through a grove of Norway spruce. Look for the bench. Take the path to your right, go down a hill, and come out on the south side of the "Wedding Meadow." Tables invite you to picnic here. It is a popular spot for weddings because all the flowering plants here have white blossoms.

➤A bench remembering "Sniffles" is on your right by the ponderosa pine at marker 8. Continue straight on Spruce Trail, crossing the Yellow Pine Trail. A sign at marker 9 gives some facts about pines, as well as a brief note about a mythological Greek goddess who reportedly cared for these trees. The beads of pitch on pine trees are said to be her tears.

➤Pass marker 9 and continue to 10. Note the two strange-looking weeping sequoias that creep along the ground by the upright ones.

➤The Spruce Trail meets the Wildwood Trail near marker 12. Turn left onto Wildwood, a popular jogging trail.

➤Go downhill through the tall sequoias of a redwood forest. A bench at the bend to the left is dedicated to two beloved dogs. A sign begins, "Go to the first star. Turn right. Head straight on till morning." Past this bench is another junction where Wildwood Trail goes downhill to the right.

➤At the junction of Wildwood and Redwood Trails, keep straight on Redwood Trail, going beneath a Port Orford cedar. Pass a bench by marker 17 and then a western redcedar. Ignore the path leading down to the creek at marker 19 and continue to the Cedar of Lebanon at marker 20.

➤You will cross another trail. Bear right to marker 22. A grassy uphill slope is on your left. Marker 24 identifies a Deodar cedar shortly before you reach SW Fischer Lane.

➤Cross SW Fischer Lane, watching carefully for traffic. Continue on the path on the other side. The memorial bench for John M. Bond is underneath a Japanese larch tree at marker 26.

➤The path goes uphill to your right through a variety of firs. You will pass a tall Noble fir, sometimes called an "Oregon Larch."

➤Go straight ahead past the junction with the Fir Trail. The picnic shelter is just ahead.

➤Turn right at the shelter and return across SW Fairview Boulevard to the visitor center.

walk 11
The Hoyt Arboretum Bristlecone Trail

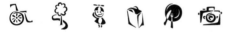

General location: Hoyt Arboretum is on the west side of Portland.

Special attractions: A sylvan retreat containing the world's largest collection of conifers.

Difficulty rating: Easy and paved. There is a slight slope.

Distance: 0.5 mile.

Estimated time: 30 minutes.

Services: The visitor center has exhibits, a horticultural library, and a small shop with tree-related gifts and books. A few snacks are also available. Drinking fountains and wheelchair-accessible restrooms are outside, along with picnic tables and a shelter.

The Hoyt Arboretum Bristlecone Trail

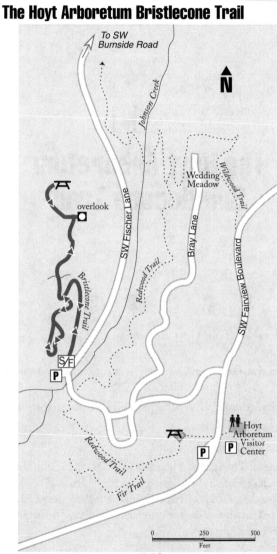

Restrictions: The wheelchair-accessible restrooms are open until the park closes at 10 P.M. The center is staffed by volunteers and is generally open each day. Visitors are prohibited from picking plants. No fires or alcoholic beverages are allowed in the park. Mountain bikes and motorized vehicles are prohibited on the trails.

For more information: Contact the Hoyt Arboretum.

Getting started: From downtown Portland, take U.S. Highway 26 westbound to the Zoo-Forestry Center exit. Follow the signs to the Hoyt Arboretum Visitor Center at 4000 SW Fairview Boulevard. You can also take Burnside Street west to the arboretum by following the entrance sign on the left about a mile west of NW 23rd. Keep following the signs to the arboretum. The main parking lot is on the south side of the visitor center.

To reach the trailhead from the arboretum parking lot, turn right onto SW Fairview Boulevard. Take the first left onto SW Fischer Lane. Drive down this lane for 0.2 miles. The parking lot for the Bristlecone Trail is on your left.

Public transportation: Bus 63 (Washington Park) from downtown Portland stops at the Hoyt Arboretum Visitor Center. Contact Tri-Met for information about fares and schedules.

Overview: This paved path takes you through a variety of conifers, with many benches and viewpoints available to help you enjoy the route.

The walk

➤A sign depicting a bristlecone pine marks the trailhead on the north side of the parking lot. Start up the trail, passing monkey puzzle trees on your left. A bench and moss-covered boulders are on your left at the top of the hill. The trail loops around a large Douglas-fir. Pacific dogwood trees are on your right.

➤Where two trails come together, take the one on your right, turning past a grand fir. A bench in memory of Martha Biggs sits by a little drainage rivulet.

➤Continue on the path past another bench in memory of Ruth Hyde and past a grove of paper birch. An overlook is on your right. From here, you can look across a little valley to a forested hill.

➤Continue to the trail's end at a picnic area.

➤Turn around and go back down the paved hill.

➤When you come to the junction of two trails at the marker for the ninebark tree, turn right. Take the path past white fir and cypress. Pass the bench by the madrone.

➤Bear right at the circle by a European white birch. You can look down at the parking lot from a bench. Then return to the trail.

➤Go down the trail to return to the parking lot.

walk **12**

Washington Park

General location: 1 mile west of downtown Portland.

Special attractions: Playgrounds, International Rose Test Gardens, Japanese Gardens, picnic tables, tennis courts. You can take a train from here to nearby Oregon Zoo.

Difficulty rating: This park is made up of a series of terraces climbing up a steep slope. You will be climbing steps, paths, or paved roads. The walk is possible with strollers, but those with wheelchairs would find the going difficult.

Distance: 2 miles through the main section of Washington Park. The side trip to the Japanese Gardens adds 1 mile.

Estimated time: 1 hour. Allow another hour for the Japanese Gardens.

Services: Water fountains and restrooms. Food is available seasonally at the kiosks at either end of the tennis courts.

Washington Park

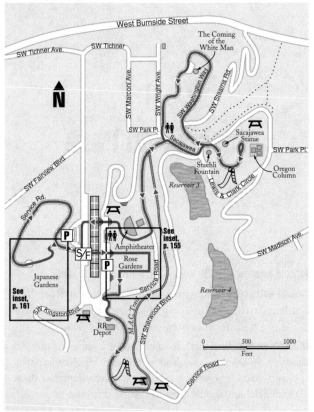

Special thanks to Portland Parks and Recreation for help with this map.

The zoo restaurant is open year-round, but you will have to pay admission to the zoo to eat there.

Restrictions: Washington Park and the International Rose Test Gardens are open daily during daylight hours. There is an admission fee to the Japanese Gardens, also open daily but hours are limited. Eating, drinking, and smoking are prohibited in the Japanese Gardens. There is limited access for the physically challenged.

For more information: Contact the Portland Oregon Visitors Association, Portland Parks and Recreation, or the Japanese Gardens.

Getting started: From Interstate 405 (northbound), take the Salmon Street exit and proceed to a left onto Burnside. From Interstate 405 (southbound), take the Burnside exit and proceed to a right onto Burnside. From either direction, take Burnside west to SW St. Clair on the left side of Burnside opposite NW 22nd Avenue. Turn left (south) onto SW St. Clair. Turn right onto SW Park Place. At the T junction, turn right to enter the park on SW Washington Way. Continue around the knoll. Several roads meet here by the reservoir. Follow the signs to the Rose and Japanese Gardens, taking Sacajawea Boulevard and Rose Garden Way up the hill to the Rose Gardens parking lot. You can park either on the Rose Garden Way or the Kingston Boulevard side of the tennis courts.

Public transportation: Tri-Met Bus 63 (Washington Park) stops at the International Rose Test Gardens, Japanese Gardens, and the Oregon Zoo. The Washington Park and Zoo Railway travels between the rose gardens and Oregon Zoo. Contact Tri-Met for information about fares and schedules.

Overview: This 332-acre park offers sweeping panoramic views, play and picnic areas, tennis courts, a zoo, and an amphitheater for outdoor concerts. It is one of Portland's oldest and best-loved parks.

Former German sailor Charles Meyers, the first park keeper, relied on his memories of European parks as he developed what was then called City Park. Former seaman Richard Knight, a Portland pharmacist, had begun purchasing the animals collected by his old shipmates during their travels. When his acquisitions outgrew his exhibition space, he donated the animals to the city for a zoo. Meyers added the role of zookeeper to his duties. He dug the first sunken bear pit in the world.

John Olmsted, of the famous firm of landscape architects, was designing parks for Seattle in 1903. During a visit to Portland, he made several suggestions for park improvements, including changing City Park's name. It became Washington Park.

The walk

➤Start this walk below the tennis courts.

➤Go through the opening in the stone wall and take the steps down to the information kiosk. Surrounded by miniature roses, the kiosk displays maps showing the park's layout and the location of each type of rose in the International Rose Test Gardens.

➤Pass the kiosk, continue on the walkway, and enjoy views of the city as you descend the steps and terraces among formal flower beds. These are test beds for roses to be selected as "All-American." They contain more than 520 varieties of roses of almost every imaginable hue—reds, lavenders, oranges, whites. They come from all over the world.

➤Continue to the overlook at the end of this garden walkway, where winning selections are displayed. The view of snow-crowned Mount Hood presiding majestically over the city shows up on many Portland posters and postcards.

➤Turn right and proceed along the Queen's Walk. Every

International Rose Test Gardens

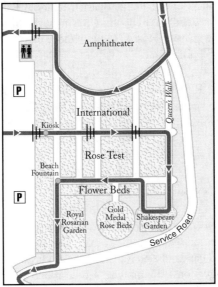

Rose Festival Queen has her name, date, and signature inscribed on a bronze tile placed on this brick walkway.

➤Continue into the Shakespeare Garden. Turn right at the center walk. Plants mentioned in Shakespeare's plays fill the boxwood-bordered flower beds.

➤Go to the bench at the far end of the garden. This bears Shakespeare's own quotation, "Of all flowres methinks a rose is best."

➤Turn right to the path exiting the garden. Proceed to the next main walkway.

➤Turn left and go up the steps under the rose trellises. The Gold Medal Test Gardens to your left contain roses especially adapted to the Northwest. Investigate these beds if you like. Then continue up to the next terrace and the stainless-steel pillars of the Frank Beach Memorial Fountain. Lee Kelly designed this in honor of the man who first called Portland the "City of Roses." Children love playing on the fountain's stepping stones.

►Turn left and walk past the fountain. You are going through the Royal Rosarian Garden, named for the civic leaders who sponsor Portland's annual Rose Festival. It is planted with their namesake roses. The Prime Minister's Walk goes around the perimeter. The Rosarians' names are inscribed on tiles.

►Continue on to the service road. Turn right to reach a junction of several roads.

►Turn left onto SW Sherwood Boulevard. Keep on the left side as you start down the hill. You will see and pass a flight of steps on the right side of road. These lead up to the Washington Park and Zoo Railway Depot. The railway carries passengers on a 35-minute, 4-mile round trip to the Oregon Zoo. This is the last official railroad in the United States to offer continual mail service. Letters deposited on the railway receive a special hand cancellation.

Two of the open-air cars have wheelchair lifts. The train runs daily from Memorial Day to Labor Day. There is a small fee to ride the train, and you must also pay for admission to the zoo. Contact the Oregon Zoo for information on rates and schedules.

►Continue walking on the left side of SW Sherwood Boulevard until you reach the children's play area. The large colorful structures here keep children busy for hours.

►Turn left into the playground. Turn right on the path toward the sandbox, then take the path on your left toward the large playhouse. A bridge connects two parts of the structure.

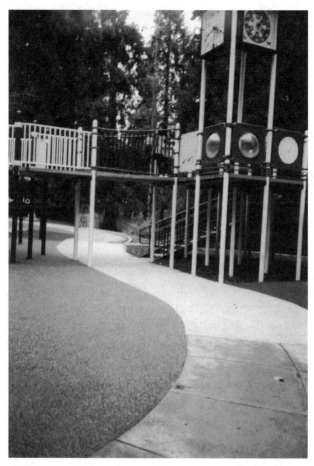

Path between two sections of the Children's Play area by the Rose gardens.

Go underneath the bridge between the blue slide and blue tunnel.

➤Turn to your right toward the stone pillar that marks a nature trail. This dirt path is the Multnomah Athletic Club (M.A.C.) Trail.

➤Continue on the trail past a little overlook. A service road is above you on the left. You will pass a small landslide, which has exposed massive and twisting tree roots. A sign on your left marks the half-mile point on the M.A.C. Trail. Below you to the right are SW Sherwood Road and a large reservoir.

➤Turn right when you come to the service road. Take this to the white posts marking its end at Sacajawea Boulevard.

➤Turn right onto Sacajawea Boulevard. Continue down the road to its junction with SW Washington Way and Lewis and Clark Circle. Wrought-iron railings and stone parapets enclose the large reservoir on your right.

➤At the center of Lewis and Clark Circle is a large grassy knoll. Cross the road to the cast-iron fountain at the base. This is the original Washington Park fountain, created in 1891 by Swiss immigrant John Staehli. Originally, a statue of a small boy, Staehli's son, stood on the top of the fountain. No one knows when or why the statue disappeared. It has never been found.

Take the path to the left of the fountain. Go to the bronze statue of Sacajawea, translator and guide to explorers Lewis and Clark. She stands on a large rock, facing west, with her infant son on her back. Women from all over the nation donated funds for this—the first public statue of a woman ever erected in the United States. Suffragists Susan B. Anthony and Abigail Scott-Duniway presided at its installation during the Lewis and Clark Centennial Exposition of 1905.

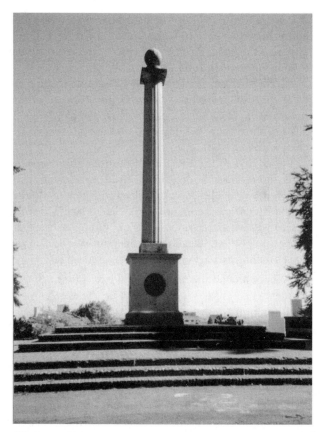

The Oregon Column.

➤Pass Sacajawea. Go up the path between a picnic area and a children's play area. Continue to the Oregon Column on top of the knoll. President Theodore Roosevelt laid the foundation stone in 1903.

Meriwether Lewis and William Clark were the first official U.S. explorers of the Oregon Country, which became the states of Oregon, Idaho, Montana, and Washington. Seals of these states are displayed on the four sides of the column's base.

Go around to the east side of the column to see how high you are above the downtown area. The steps in front of you go down to a brick wall crowned with flowers, Washington Park's formal entrance on SW Park Place. The street descends down a steep slope into the city. It makes you realize how important Staehli's fountain must have been to the horses pulling carriages full of visitors up this hill.

➤Go back around the memorial and return to the Staehli fountain.

➤Turn right onto SW Washington Way.

➤Continue on Washington Way around the knoll, passing by the entrance to SW Stearns Road. You will come to a small parking pullout. Another bronze sculpture, entitled *The Coming of the White Man*, is on the knoll.

➤Turn left and go up the knoll for a closer look at the statue. A young brave is showing Chief Multnomah some explorers coming down the Willamette River.

The family of former Portland mayor David Thompson asked sculptor Herman McNeil to create this gift to the city in 1904. He chose this subject because he had been fascinated by Indians ever since seeing Buffalo Bill's Wild West show. McNeil visited several Indian reservations while doing his research, and he supposedly modeled the older man after the real Chief Multnomah.

Japanese Gardens

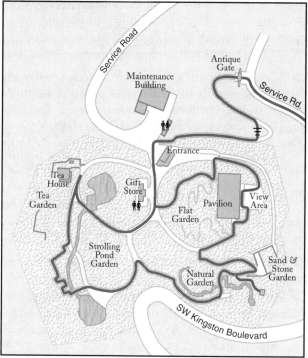

➤Continue around SW Washington Way to the small brick restroom building.

➤Cross Sacajawea Boulevard to the service road. Turn right onto this road.

➤Continue past the 0.3-mile marker on the M.A.C. Trail until you come to a walkway on your right.

➤Turn right onto this walkway. The amphitheater on your right is used for summer outdoor concerts. The International Rose Test Gardens are on your left.

161

➤Continue on this walkway until you reach a T junction. Turn right and continue until you see a flight of steps on your left.

➤Go up these steps to Rose Garden Way. (There will be a restroom on your left.)

➤Cross the road, go up more steps between the tennis courts to SW Kingston Boulevard. On the other side of the road is a small parking area for the Japanese Gardens.

The Japanese Garden Society of Oregon began creating these gardens in 1962. Designed by landscape architect Professor Takuma Tono of Tokyo Agricultural University, they are considered the most beautiful and authentic landscape of this type outside Japan. There is an admission charge. If you decide to enter, cross the road into the parking lot, turn left, and follow the sign pointing to the Japanese Gardens.

➤Turn right on the road.

➤Turn left at the antique gate and take the path to the main entrance.

➤After paying the entrance fee and getting a map, walk through the ceramic-tiled entrance gate. In less than a mile, you will walk through five different landscapes, each with its own distinct mood. The sound of water from fountains and waterfalls encourages slow strolling, quiet conversation, and frequent pauses. Each garden provides many changing views and is beautiful in every season of the year. The pink and white blossoms of the cherry trees unfold each spring, the Japanese maples display every possible shade of red or orange in autumn, and the gardens' evergreens add to the tranquility of winter.

Many paths have uneven surfaces, making the gardens difficult to explore for those who are physically challenged. In the Natural Garden, stone steps take you up and down

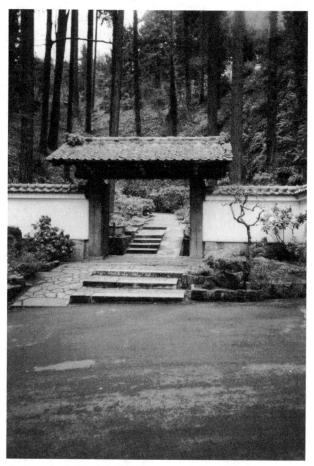

Antique gate in Japanese Gardens.

along waterscapes with small ponds, streams, and water-falls. These can be slippery. Some of the pools are deep, and all are unprotected. Watch your children and your footing at all times as you navigate this particular area.

The Strolling Pond Garden has two sections. Crane sculptures and an authentic Moon Bridge are major features of the Upper Pond. The golden koi fish in the Lower Pond seem to enjoy people watching as much as the people do. A wooden bridge takes you through iris beds and across the pond.

Weathered stones rise from sand raked carefully into wavelike patterns in the Sand and Stone Garden, while the sand in the Flat Garden resembles Japanese floor matting. Pleasure and happiness are symbolized by two mossy green plantings shaped like a saki bottle and a gourd bottle.

There are two Tea Gardens—an outer one where one waits for the tea ceremony, and an inner one surrounding the "Flower Heart" ceremonial tea house. A gift store at the entrance contains gifts, restrooms, and a drinking fountain.

➤Leave the garden through the gate. Return down the path to your starting point in the parking area.

walk **13**

Council Crest

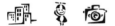

General location: Marquam Hill in southwest Portland, near the Doernbecher, Shriners, Veterans Administration, and Oregon Health Sciences University Hospitals.

Special attractions: Scenic views from Council Crest, the highest point in Portland (1,070 feet).

Difficulty rating: Difficult. The first leg of the walk is on a short and steep dirt trail. Fairmont Boulevard is flat and paved but has no shoulders.

Distance: 4.5 miles.

Estimated time: 3 hours.

Services: There are restrooms and water in Council Crest Park on top of the hill.

Restrictions: When walking on the road, be sure to walk single file facing traffic. The Fairmont Boulevard "linear park"

Council Crest

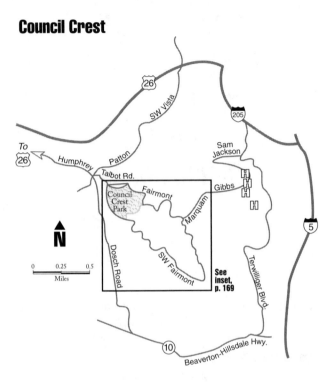

circles Council Crest Hill, and the road is shared by motorists, bicyclists, walkers, and runners.

For more information: Contact Portland Parks and Recreation.

Getting started: The walk begins at the Council Crest Trailhead at the junction of SW Talbot Road and Fairmont Boulevard. From Interstate 405 southbound, take the 6th Avenue exit and follow the blue hospital signs. Turn right onto 6th, which becomes Terwilliger Boulevard. This is only the first of many name changes this road undergoes as it ascends Council Crest Hill.

Continue straight on Terwilliger past Duniway Park and a service station on the left side of the road. The Carnival Restaurant on your right is a good place to stop for refreshments before or after your walk. The road is now called Sam Jackson Park Road. Continue on this road as it skirts Doernbecher Hospital, and then keep to the right on Gibbs Road as it goes between the Oregon Health Sciences University (OHSU) Hospital and the University of Oregon Dental School. Follow Gibbs, which becomes Marquam Hill Road, to the T intersection at Fairmont. Turn right onto Fairmont and proceed to the intersection with Talbot Road. There is a parking area at the trailhead. Parking is also permitted along the sides of the road.

Public transportation: Tri-Met Bus 51 (Council Crest) goes to SW Talbot at Greenway. Contact Tri-Met for information about schedules and fares.

Overview: This short section of Marquam Trail takes you up through deep woods to Council Crest, the highest point in Portland. You will have a gorgeous view of the city, the Willamette River, and the mountains beyond. An outdoor observation circle shows compass directions and identifies the mountains. The Marquam Trail takes you back down the hill to Fairmont from the other side of the knoll.

Fairmont is a fine residential neighborhood, noted for its homes with spectacular views. Being one of the relatively few flat areas in this part of Portland, it attracts runners and bicyclists. Most drivers watch out for pedestrian traffic, but make sure you keep to the side of the road and face oncoming cars.

The walk

➤The walk begins at the trailhead parking area at the junction of Fairmont and Talbot. Start at the sign reading "Marquam Trail." You are 0.3 mile from Council Crest Park and 2 miles from the Marquam Nature Shelter.

➤Step over the logs at the trailhead and follow the trail a short distance to the post at the Y intersection. Take the left-hand trail to Council Crest. The trail is steep here as it goes uphill through the woods. Tall Douglas-fir, Western hemlock, and bigleaf maples line the trail.

➤Just before you come out of the woods, you can see the metal legs of a TV tower. The trail ends at a sidewalk.

➤Follow this sidewalk up to the road. Restrooms are in the brick building on your left under the tower.

➤Turn to your right on the road and continue to the bench near a lovely bronze sculpture. You will have an incredible view of the Tualatin Valley.

The unusual sculptured fountain was donated by Florence and George Laboree. It was created by Frederic Littman, who also created the *Farewell to Orpheus* fountain at Portland State University. Water flows from flower-shaped spouts, while the figures of a mother and child show pure delight in each other. Littman hammered and welded the bronze in such a way that the entire piece seems to balance on the mother's toe.

➤Cross the road toward the water tower. Climb the grassy knoll. This is a green, lovely, and tranquil place at the zenith of the city. A visitor whose spouse was staying in a nearby hospital noted that she could "just feel the stress pouring off up here."

Council Crest

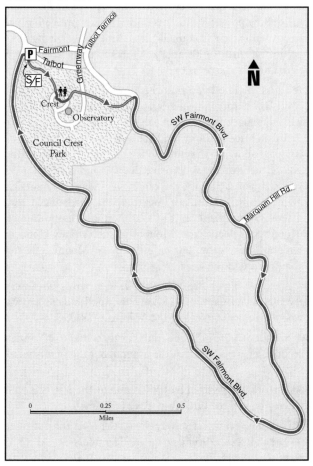

N

Fairmont

Talbot

Talbot Terrace

Greenway

P

S/F

Crest

Observatory

Council Crest
Park

SW Fairmont Blvd

Marquam Hill Rd.

SW Fairmont Blvd.

0   0.25   0.5
Miles

Council Crest Park was named by a group of Congregational ministers and their wives who were picnicking here in 1898. Supposedly, this was once a meeting place for Native American tribal councils. It became accessible by cable car in the early 1900s and was the site of an amusement park until the Depression.

➤Cross the knoll and find the observation circle, a round courtyard bordered by a brick wall. Anything you say here will come back to you as an echo.

Inlaid brick in the ground has been used to depict a large compass showing the directions and degrees between the points. Signs on the walls make this a "mountain finder." As you gaze across the city, you can easily find each mountain's name, height, and distance from this point on Council Crest. There are wonderful views of Washington's Mount Rainier, Mount St. Helens, and Mount Adams. Mount Hood in Oregon is also clear, but only the tip of Mount Jefferson shows through the trees.

➤The next leg of the Marquam Trail is across Greenway Avenue from this point. Go down the knoll and cross to the wooden signpost marking the Marquam Trail.

➤Start down the hill. The trail quickly comes to a Y intersection. There is a post in the ground, but the sign is missing.

➤Turn to the right. The trail bends to the left at a spot where you can see Greenway Avenue below.

➤Continue on to Greenway. Cross the road and continue on the trail as it descends on a gentle grade.

➤The next road you meet is Fairmont Boulevard. Although Marquam Trail continues across the road, you will stay on Fairmont.

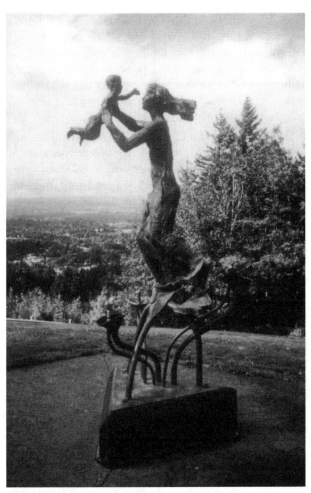

Ode to Joy sculpture and fountain.

(*Author's note:* Since Fairmont makes a complete 3.8-mile loop around Council Crest, you have two options here. If you are ready to stop, you can turn left and take the 0.8-mile walk back to your starting point. Keep on Fairmont to Talbot Road and take a left under the Greenway overpass to return to the trailhead. If you want to continue walking, proceed with the following directions.)

➤Turn to your right for a 3-mile walk through the Fairmont neighborhood. This residential area was developed early in the century and was the site of one of Portland's first scenic drives. The older homes are tucked away on the many secluded drives angling from the road. More modern houses roost on small hillside terraces or are propped precariously on stilts.

Fairmont follows a contour line around the hill, so you get many different glimpses of the city through the trees as you circle back to your starting point.

➤Look for the large blue hospital sign to point your way back to the city. The street sign for Marquam Road is hidden by foliage. As you descend this steep hill, known as "Pill Hill" because of the hospitals, you may see Bus 8 (Jackson) making its stops. A friend was riding this bus one day when a man in a wheelchair bet the other passengers he could beat the bus to the bottom of the hill. When a few put up some money, he got off the bus and raced his wheelchair to the bottom, easily beating the bus, which had more stops to make. After he had collected his winnings and the passengers had settled back into their seats, the driver looked around with a wide smile and said, "He always wins!" It's a good story, though the road seems far too narrow for wheelchair racing. Still, you may want to beware of speeding wheelchairs as you drop down into the city.

walk 14

Tryon Creek State Park

General location: Southwest Portland, east of Interstate 5.

Special attractions: Nature, hiking, and equestrian trails through a beautiful second-growth forest.

Difficulty rating: The first part of the walk is on the Trillium Trail, an easy, paved, completely wheelchair-accessible path. By 1998 this trail will also be accessible to those with visual difficulties, with changing textures in the pavement signaling the availability of recorded descriptive information. Ask at the Nature Center for these tape recorders. The remainder of the trail is difficult because it is on dirt paths with many ups and downs.

Distance: 3 miles.

Estimated time: 2 hours.

Services: Wildlife exhibits, water, wheelchair-accessible restrooms, small gift shop with an excellent selection of books on natural history.

Restrictions: Open dawn to dusk daily. The paved, wheel-chair-accessible Trillium Trail is 0.35-mile long before it rejoins the Old Main Trail by the nature center. Pets must be kept on a 6-foot-maximum leash at all times, and their droppings must be removed. Bicyclists are restricted to the paved bike trail, and horseback riders must stay in a single file on designated equestrian trails. Walkers should stay on the trail at all times. Take only photographs—do not disturb the plants or animals—and leave only footprints.

For more information: Contact Tryon Creek State Park or the Nature House.

Getting started: This walk begins at the Nature Center in Tryon Creek State Park, which is about 2.5 miles from Interstate 5.

From I-5 southbound, take the Exit 297, Terwilliger Boulevard, and cross the freeway on the overpass. From I-5 northbound, take the Exit 297, Terwilliger Boulevard. From either direction, drive south on Terwilliger through the intersection with Taylors Ferry Road. At the traffic light at the intersection with Boones Ferry Road, bear left, then bear right at the next intersection to continue on Terwilliger toward Lake Oswego. You will pass the entrance to the Lewis and Clark Law School. The entrance to the park will be down the road about a mile on your right.

Public transportation: From Burlingame Transit Center, Bus 39 stops at Lewis and Clark College. Contact Tri-Met for information about schedules and fares.

Overview: *Forest in a City*, a guidebook published by the Friends of Tryon Creek State Park, points out that this park represents several "firsts" in the Oregon parks system. It was the first state park established within a city's limits, the first

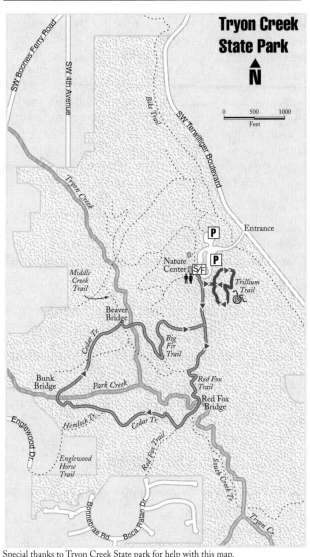

Tryon Creek
State Park

N

SW Boones Ferry Road

SW 4th Avenue

Bike Trail

SW Terwilliger Boulevard

0   500   1000
Feet

Tryon Creek

Entrance

P

P

Nature
Center

S/F

Trillium
Trail

*Middle
Creek
Trail*

Beaver
Bridge

Cedar Tr.

*Big
Fir
Trail*

Bunk
Bridge

Park Creek

*Red Fox
Trail*

Red Fox
Bridge

Hemlock Tr.

Cedar Tr.

Red Fox Trail

Englewood Dr.

*Englewood
Horse
Trail*

South Creek Tr.

Tryon Cr.

Bonnebrae Rd.

Boca Ratan Dr.

Special thanks to Tryon Creek State park for help with this map.

with a master plan, the first to encourage citizen involvement from the beginning, the first to have a nature center, and the first to have a trail accessible by all.

The Friends of Tryon Creek State Park worked hard to ensure that this area would become a state park rather than a housing development. They raised enough money to buy the property in the early 1970s and then lobbied state officials and Governor Tom McCall to create it. They also designed and built the award-winning Nature Center. This active group provides staffing for special programs and events and some of the maintenance necessary for the park's operations.

Tryon Creek State Park changes with the seasons but is always a lush retreat. It is well known for its profusion of trilliums in the spring, and it hosts a Trillium Festival each April. Park volunteers offer guided hikes on occasional weekdays and some weekends. The Nature Center, open daily, has exhibits on park history, vegetation, and wildlife.

This walk is primarily along the natural trails and asphalt paths winding through this ever-changing second-growth forest. Birdsong and the chirrups of small animals are constant reminders of the 120 species that call this park home.

Before starting this walk, browse through the Nature Center and take a good look at the large relief map near the door to the back deck. The exhibits and map provide a good introduction to the park.

The walk

➤Start this walk at the kiosk in the parking lot outside the Nature Center.

➤Take the path to your left marked "Nature Trail." You will see a dispenser for dog-waste scoops.

➤Follow the signs to the entrance of the Trillium Trail. This is an all-abilities paved trail with two small loops. Its total length is 0.35 mile. Notice the different textures in the pavement under your feet. These changing surfaces are signals to those with visual problems to turn on the recorders provided by the Nature Center and listen to descriptions of the surroundings.

Note signs marking the site of an old logging road. The planting of native trees and shrubs has almost obscured this mark of man and restored a more natural setting.

➤Follow the sign indicating the upper loop of the trail. The next marker is at one of the few spots where sunlight actually reaches the forest floor. The sign points out that, as the trees keep growing, shade-loving plants eventually will replace the present sun-loving plants. There is a bench and water fountain here.

➤Go to the overlook deck and look down into the bottom of a deep ravine. Then continue on to the T intersection.

➤Take the lower loop of the Trillium Trail. The next sign points out old stumps remaining from the original firs and cedars that were logged between the 1880s and 1920s. These trees eventually became lumber and charcoal for a nearby iron smelter. You will pass another overlook with a different view of the ravine. You can sit and use all your senses to experience the surrounding forest.

The next marker gives some history of the park. The only reason this forest will continue to grow is because the Friends of Tryon Creek State Park protected the area from development.

➤Take the bark-covered Old Main Trail to your left. The woodsy scent of the forest surrounds you as you walk along the trail under a canopy of Douglas-fir and bigleaf maples.

177

This is a typical Western Oregon forest, with moss-covered branches, trees, and stumps. Ferns are abundant.

There is a bench in an open spot at the junction of Old Main, Big Fir, and Red Fox Trails. This spot has a good view of Tryon Creek Canyon.

➤Turn to your left onto Red Fox Trail, which goes down a rather steep hill and continues to the left around a tall Douglas-fir. Western redcedars are on either side. You can also see clusters of Oregon grape, with the hollylike leaves and yellow flowers that will become blue, sour berries by late summer. The trail bends around, bringing you to the bottom of the canyon.

The rustic Red Fox Bridge crosses Tryon Creek. If you want to have a close look at the creek, take the steps that lead down to it. Then return to the footbridge and cross.

➤The trail continues uphill on the other side. This part of the trail has several ups and downs as it goes through a grove of red alders.

➤Pass the junction with South Creek Trail and continue uphill to your right. An old tree stump riddled with oblong holes made by pileated woodpeckers is on the right-hand side of the trail. On the left is a clump of bracken ferns. As you continue uphill, log posts border the trail. At the top of the hill, a sign reads "Red Fox Trail."

➤You will take the Cedar Trail. Loop around to your right to find it. You can certainly see how this trail got its name. Tall western redcedars surround you and seem to meet overhead. You can hear the wind in the trees and birds singing from the treetops.

This part of the walk goes uphill on gravel. Notice the English ivy spreading across the slopes to the left and right. This ivy escaped from neighboring gardens and can deprive the native plants of food, water, and sunlight. It can eventually strangle any tree it climbs. There is an "adopt-a-plot" ivy-removal program under way.

➤A boardwalk on the path takes you safely across a swampy area. Continue to a larger footbridge and cross. Notice the water-smoothed boulder lying in the little rivulet that comes down from the left, as well as the moss-covered cedar with roots almost out of the ground. Lady ferns cluster around the path. At the top of the slope is a marker telling you that Beaver Bridge is to the left and Red Fox Bridge is to the right.

➤Continue on Cedar Trail, passing markers for both Hemlock Trail and Englewood Drive. The narrow hard-packed dirt trail winds among red alders and around a lovely little nursery stump with small plants sprouting from its top.

➤Take Bunk Bridge over Park Creek. The trail turns to the right and then climbs over some twisted roots that act as steps.

➤Cross another muddy area on a boardwalk. You are now in a grove where many of the trees have ferns sprouting from their sides. Note the large tree with a damaged center section. The branches continue to grow upward, while ferns grow out of the entire lower part of the tree.

➤You will soon come to a spot where many trails meet. A post in the center of the intersection is surrounded by signs. The first sign on your left is for an equestrian trail going to West Horse Loop and Englewood Drive. The next shows a horseshoe with a red bar through it and a footprint. This is the Cedar Trail to Beaver Bridge. On your right is a sign that reads "West Equestrian Loop."

➤Take the Cedar Trail to Beaver Bridge. There are steps here that are absolutely essential for safety, since this path down to Tryon Creek is slippery.

➤Follow the sign marked with a footprint and continue on the path across the West Horse Loop. You will see a sign for Middle Creek Trail. High Bridge is to your left, and Beaver Bridge and the Nature Center are to the right. Listen to the chatter of the tree squirrels in the stillness here.

➤Cross over Beaver Bridge. Look down the canyon to see Obie's Bridge.

➤Go across the boardwalk. At the top of the slope, where Big Fir Trail joins the path, is another bench where you can sit and catch your breath.

➤At the junction where the trails go left and right, take the left-hand Big Fir Trail back to the junction with Old Main Trail. This is a more open section of the park, with ferns covering the ground and alders lining the trail.

➤Turn left onto Old Main Trail and follow the arrow back to the Nature Center.

walk 15

Powell Butte Nature Park

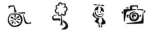

General location: Southeast Portland, about 5 miles east of Interstate 205.

Special attractions: About 570 acres of Douglas-fir forest and upland meadows, with magnificent views of the mountains and city from the 630-foot summit of Powell Butte. This park is considered one of the 20 best sites for birders in the Portland area, with lazuli buntings, barn owls, and northern shrike among the species you might see here.

Difficulty rating: Moderate. The paved 0.6-mile path to the top of the 630-foot butte has switchbacks for wheelchair accessibility. The remainder of the walk is on a narrow dirt path.

Distance: About 3 miles.

Estimated time: 1.5 hours.

Services: Wheelchair-accessible restrooms, water fountain, picnic area.

Powell Butte Nature Park

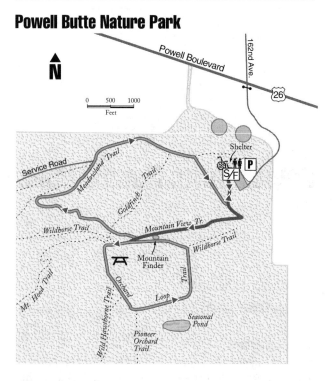

Restrictions: The park is open from dawn to dusk. No motorized vehicles of any kind are permitted beyond the parking area. Dogs must be leashed and their droppings removed. Alcohol, firearms, open camping, golfing, and vending are prohibited. To help prevent erosion, please stay on the officially designated trails.

For more information: Contact the Friends of Powell Butte or Portland Parks and Recreation.

Getting started: To reach the park entrance at the intersection of Powell Boulevard and 162nd Avenue from the west

182

side of Portland, take U.S. Highway 26 across the Ross Island Bridge. On the east side of the bridge, the road becomes Powell Boulevard. To reach the park entrance from Interstate 205, take the Division Street exit. Go east to 162nd Avenue, turn right, and take 162nd south to Powell Boulevard. Cross Powell. Meadow Crest Farm Estates will be on your left, and there should be a sign reading "Welcome to Powell Butte Nature Park." Follow the road uphill half a mile to the parking lot.

Public transportation: Take Bus 9 (Powell/Gresham) to the park. Contact Tri-Met for information about fares and schedules.

Overview: Powell Butte is an old shield volcano and former farm. In the 1920s, the City of Portland purchased this land to use for water reservoirs and built a 50-million-gallon underground tank. There is room for four more. The dairy farm functioned until 1948, and cattle continued grazing until 1990, when it became a nature park.

The park is home to many species of wildlife. As you walk, you may see coyotes, squirrels, raccoons, rabbits, and deer. You may see hawks flying over the meadows and hear meadowlarks and sparrows singing in the orchards, shrubs, and thickets along the trail.

There are 9 miles of trail for hiking, horseback riding, and mountain biking. This particular walk takes you on two intersecting loop trails. One is at the top of the butte, where you will have views of 15 hills and mountains, and the other is through a meadow at the butte's base.

The walk

➤The walk begins at the shelter at the Powell Butte parking area. The signboard opposite the restrooms displays a map of the trails, as well as information about the park's history and the different flora and fauna. There is a picnic table here.

➤Exit this area on the paved path to your left. This is Mountain View Trail, a 0.6-mile, wheelchair-accessible trail that has many switchbacks in its 5-percent uphill grade. There are level rest stops every 200 feet.

A concrete-lined culvert collects rainwater and is a reminder of the reservoir underground. As you climb upward, you will be surrounded by wildflowers, hawthorn bushes, thistles, and wild blackberries. Just after the path makes a left turn, you will cross the Meadowland Trail and a service road.

➤Continue on the paved path to the top of the hill. The paving ends at the summit, where the path joins Orchard Loop Trail.

➤Turn right onto Orchard Loop Trail, which makes a complete loop around the summit. It is open to horseback riders, as well as bicyclists and hikers, so watch your step!

On your left are apple, pear, and filbert trees—remnants of the farm that originally occupied this site. Though no longer cultivated or sprayed, the trees are in full bloom during springtime and provide fruit for the butte's wildlife.

➤The Orchard Loop Trail makes a sharp left after it crosses the Wildhorse and Mount Hood Trails.

➤Continue down the hill, enjoying the silence of your surroundings.

➤The trail bends left just after the junction with Pioneer Orchard Trail. Now you are going uphill on Orchard Loop Trail. Down the hill to your right is a fenced-off seasonal pond that provides water for the resident wildlife.

➤When you see the city of Gresham spread out in front of you, take the first left. The path continues across a rocky area.

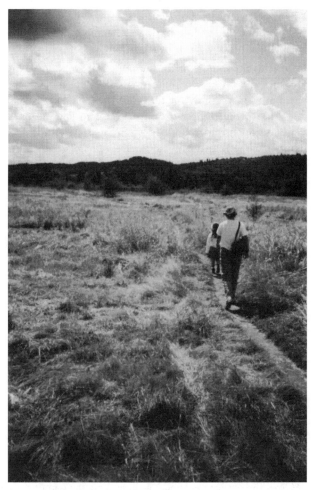

Walking Orchard Trail in Powell Butte Nature Park.
PHOTO BY ROBERT S. COOK

➤Turn left at the end of the road, cross Wildhorse Trail, and continue up the hill. Spring and summer wildflowers are abundant in these brushy old meadows.

➤Once again you are at the summit, with good views of Portland and Gresham. You can even see the smoke from paper mills in Washington, far across the Columbia River.

Look to your right and spot the old logs laid out on a gravel circle on the ground. This is a "mountain finder." It points out the four major mountains—Hood, Adams, St. Helens, and Jefferson—and many hills that you can see on clear days. It also shows the degrees of the compass used to locate hills and mountains from this point and gives the distances to each.

➤Continue west past the picnic table to paved Mountain View Trail.

➤Start down the hill on Mountain View Trail. In only a few feet, you will come to the intersection of Meadowland Trail. Turn left onto Meadowland, a trail only for hikers and bikers. The dirt path makes a few small bends to the left and right as it continues down the hill and winds through the grasslands.

➤Where it crosses a small unsigned cutoff to Cedar Grove Trail, Meadowland Trail turns sharply to the right, making almost a hairpin turn. Keep on Meadowland.

➤You will pass another junction with Cedar Grove Trail going off to the left into the trees. Continue straight north across the meadow. The trail becomes open to horses as it is joined by Wildhorse Trail.

➤Cross the service road and continue. The trail comes close to the park border and then bends to the right.

➤Continue straight to the second junction with Wildhorse Trail. Take Wildhorse Trail back to the parking lot.

walk 16

Crystal Springs and Johnson Creek

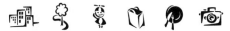

General location: Southeast Portland, 5 miles east of downtown and 12 miles south of the airport.

Special attractions: Natural wetlands and creek, a college campus, and gardens surrounding a spring-fed lake. Crystal Springs Rhododendron Garden is wheelchair accessible.

Difficulty rating: Moderate. Mostly flat, on sidewalks or dirt trails.

Distance: About 2.5 miles.

Estimated time: 2 hours.

Services: Restrooms and water are available at the trailhead parking lot, Reed College, and Crystal Springs Rhododendron Garden.

Crystal Springs and Johnson Creek

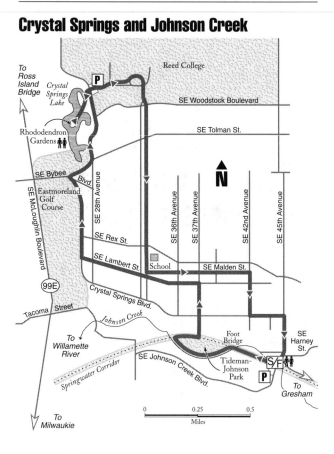

Restrictions: Crystal Springs Rhododendron Garden is open dawn to dusk seven days a week. There is a $2 admission fee for adults during the summer, from Thursday through Monday, 10 A.M. to 6 P.M. Other hours and days are free. Dogs must be leashed and their droppings picked up.

For more information: Contact Portland Parks and Recreation, Friends of Johnson Creek, or Friends of the Crystal Springs Rhododendron Garden.

Getting started: The walk begins at the Springwater Corridor Trailhead on SE 45th Avenue and SE Johnson Creek Boulevard. To reach the trailhead from Interstate 5, take the Ross Island Bridge exit, cross the bridge, and go east on Powell Boulevard (U.S. Highway 26) to SE 39th Avenue. Turn right on 39th, go south to Woodstock, and turn left. Go straight on Woodstock to 45th. Turn right on 45th, which will become Johnson Creek Boulevard after it crosses SE Harney Street.

Watch for the yellow sign alerting motorists to pedestrians and bicyclists, just before you come to the bridge over Johnson Creek. Cross the bridge and turn right into the first driveway immediately past the bridge and before the driveway for Associated Chemists, Inc. This is the Creek Trail parking lot at the Springwater Corridor Trailhead. There are picnic tables, wheelchair-accessible restrooms, and water here.

Public transportation: From downtown, take Bus 19 (Woodstock) to 45th and Woodstock. Transfer to Bus 75 (39th Avenue) and take this to 45th at Johnson Creek. Bus 19 (Woodstock) also stops at the front entrance to Reed College. Contact Tri-Met for information about fares and schedules.

Overview: This walk through the Eastmoreland area takes you through many different environments. The 18-mile-long Springwater Corridor Trail is located on an abandoned railroad line and goes east from here to Gresham and Boring. It provides access to wildlife areas, wetlands, and parks. It also joins the 40-Mile Loop—actually about 140 miles now—intended to circle Portland and link every park in the city-park system. The trail is clearly marked with mile markers.

189

Johnson Creek, an urban stream, flows 24 miles before emptying into the Willamette River. Along its banks is Tideman-Johnson Park, a natural wetland and home to great horned and screech owls. The donors of this park still live on the south side of the creek.

A completely different type of wildlife refuge is found in Crystal Springs Rhododendron Garden. In 1950, the American Rhododendron Society began transforming this unused, blackberry-infested, brushy area into a test garden for new rhododendrons. It is now a Portland showplace, especially lovely in spring and summer when the rhododendrons and azaleas are in full bloom. All of the plants have been given by interested individuals, and funds were donated to create the three waterfalls. Rhododendron Society volunteers and Master Gardeners take care of the plants, while Portland Parks and Recreation maintains lawns and restrooms.

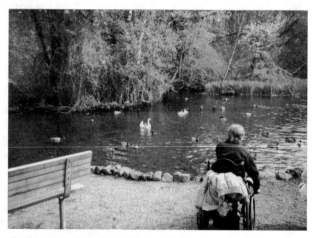

Feeding the ducks in Crystal Springs Lake.

Reed College is one of the nation's most prestigious private colleges, well known for its outstanding liberal-arts program. The original 86 acres of the campus, along with the area occupied by the rhododendron garden, was once part of Crystal Springs Farm. Few trees were here when the college was founded. Many of the lovely old trees gracing the campus today were collected from other parts of Oregon by W. F. Eliot, who donated them to the college. Reed is near the extensive and beautiful Eastmoreland Golf Course and is surrounded by beautifully maintained old homes.

The walk

➤ Go through the barriers and head west on the Springwater Trail as it enters the Johnson Creek Watershed.

➤ Continue over the wooden footbridge spanning Johnson Creek. Just past the bridge, a dirt path leads off to the left.

➤ Take this path down into Tideman-Johnson Nature Park. The path curves along the north bank of Johnson Creek. Many hard-working volunteers are removing the blackberries that have taken over the riverbank and are replanting the area with the shrubs and grasses that formerly inhabited the area. Passersby can now see the creek and have a better chance of seeing the variety of plants and animals that live in and along this urban stream. Owls live here but are rarely seen during the day.

➤ Follow the path along the creek, under the wooden bridge, and up to the main Springwater Trail.

➤ Turn right onto the Springwater.

➤ Continue east to the open area with a large sign on your right. This sign gives information about the entire Johnson Creek Watershed and its indigenous wildlife.

➤Turn around and face away from the sign. You can see a path going up the hill. Take this to the yellow metal gate.

➤You are at the foot of SE 37th Avenue. Continue north on this street. You are walking on broken pavement.

➤Proceed north for four blocks to SE Lambert Street, crossing Crystal Springs Blvd., Nehalem, and Lexington Streets.

➤Turn left onto Lambert. Continue for four blocks to Reed College Place. This street has a tree-lined parkway down its center. Note the well-preserved old elms.

➤Cross Reed College Place to its west side and cross to the north side of Lambert. Turn left and continue on Lambert for six more blocks. The houses underneath the old maples and chestnut trees seem like comfortable family homes.

➤Cross SE 28th Avenue and go down the hill to the yield sign at SE 27th Avenue.

➤Turn right. The houses along 27th have beautifully maintained lawns and shrubs.

➤Walk to SE Rex Street, where there are stop signs. Cross 27th to the sidewalk along the iron fence of the golf course. The Eastmoreland Golf Course, one of the first golf courses in Portland, was part of the original plan for the area.

➤Continue along this sidewalk until you reach SE Bybee Boulevard. The parking areas for the golf course are at the junction of Bybee and Tolman Streets. Cross Bybee with care. There are no stop signs here. The sidewalk and your route follow the golf course fence to the right as it curves around a corner and continues north along 28th Avenue.

Across the road you can see Carlton, Martins, and Moreland Streets. SE Woodstock Boulevard is next. The golf course ends here, and Crystal Springs Rhododendron Garden begins. You can see the park on your left.

➤Continue on SE 28th Avenue to the Crystal Springs Rhododendron Garden parking lot and entrance. These gardens are well worth a visit. They are beautiful year-round but are especially gorgeous in the springtime, when the flowering trees and plants are blooming. The park is almost completely surrounded by water and has several small waterfalls.

➤Enter the park by the new gatehouse and viewing terrace. Go down the paved walk. Tall rhododendrons and azalea bushes with flowers of all colors surround you. Notice the gorgeous Japanese cherry tree on your right as you proceed down to Crystal Springs Lake and its small rocky waterfall. Bridges span the lake.

➤Keep on the main path to the duck-feeding area. Crystal Springs Lake is a winter home to a variety of waterfowl. You can usually see ruddy ducks, wood ducks, buffleheads, and canvasbacks here, along with the ubiquitous mallards.

➤If you wish to spend more time in this park, take the causeway across the lake to the small island straight ahead.

➤The main path on the island will take you to the exhibit hall. Go around this building and pass the high fountain. Restrooms are off to your left.

➤Proceed on the road past the fountain to the lawn. This is a favorite spot for outdoor weddings. The large Cynthia rhododendrons edging the lawn on the west side were the first ones planted in this park.

➤After exploring the gardens, return to the causeway and take the main path back to the entrance.

➤Cross the parking lot to SE 28th Avenue. Cross 28th. Enter the west parking lot of Reed College.

➤Cross the lot to the map of the campus. Look for the walkways passing the Prexy Building, the Old Dorm Block, and Eliot Hall. If you feel like a snack, you can find one in the Commons Building, just north of the dorms. A coffee shop and campus bookstore are inside.

➤Follow the walkways through the campus. After you pass Eliot, turn right onto the college drive. The Douglas-fir here was one of the original old trees on Crystal Springs Farm. Take this drive south, past the pillar marking Reed College, to SE Woodstock Boulevard.

➤Take the crosswalk on your left. Cars must obey a stop sign, but be careful. Cross, turn right, and go to Reed College Place.

➤Turn south onto this street, keeping on the sidewalk on the east (left) side of the street. This well-maintained college neighborhood has a traditional feel. The elms in the parkway down the center are survivors of the Dutch elm epidemic that decimated trees throughout the United States. Imagine what this parkway must have looked like when it was filled with tall trees spreading a canopy across the streets.

➤Cross SE Tolman Street and walk four blocks to SE Rex Street, passing Claybourne, Bybee, and Knapp.

➤Cross Rex. The classically designed school on this corner was named for Abigail Scott-Duniway, an early Oregon leader of the women's rights movement. The school was once surrounded by lawns, which have since been replaced by blacktop play and parking areas.

➤Continue past the school to SE Malden Street and cross.

➤Turn left onto Malden and continue east for three long blocks until you reach SE 42nd Avenue.

➤Turn right onto 42nd and continue south for four blocks to Crystal Springs Boulevard.

➤Turn left onto Crystal Springs Boulevard. Cross 42nd. Continue straight to SE 45th Avenue, a busy commercial street.

➤Turn right onto 45th and continue downhill on a dirt path.

➤Take 45th south for three blocks to SE Harney Street.

➤Cross Harney at the signal and proceed to your starting point in the parking lot.

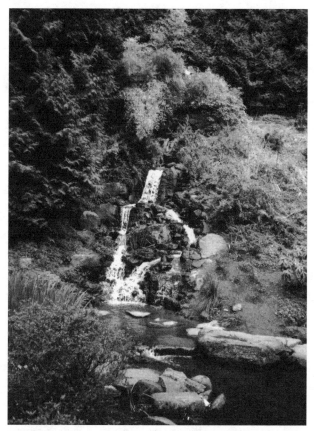

The Floweree Waterfalls Garden. PHOTO BY FRANCES CORCORAN

195

walk **17**

Mount Tabor Park

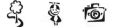

General location: The east side of Portland, south of Interstate 84 and east of Interstate 5.

Special attractions: Walk on top of the only extinct volcanic cinder cone in the center of a U.S. city. There are natural areas, reservoirs, and views of Portland.

Difficulty rating: Moderate, with one hill. Entirely on paved roads. Although the walk is suitable for strollers, it is quite steep and many areas are not accessible to wheelchairs.

Distance: 2 miles.

Estimated time: 1 hour.

Services: Parking and portable toilets; covered picnic shelter; playground; basketball, volleyball, and tennis courts.

Restrictions: Portland enforces its scoop law. Dogs must be leashed to and from the off-leash areas, and their droppings must be disposed of.

Mount Tabor Park

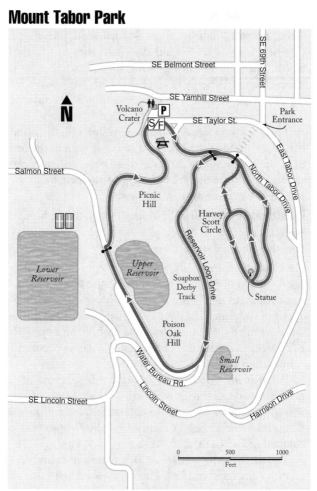

Special thanks to Portland Parks and Recreation for help with this map.

197

For more information: Contact Portland Parks and Recreation.

Getting started: From Interstate 84 eastbound, take Exit 5, Oregon Highway 213 (82nd Avenue), south to SE Stark Street. Go right (west) on Stark, following the signs to Mount Tabor. When you reach SE 69th Avenue, go left (south) straight into the park, and turn right onto SE Taylor Street.

There is a sign for pedestrians regarding a flight of steps that leads up into the park. If you are walking into the park from the bus stop, you can take these steps, and then turn right onto Taylor Street at the top of the first flight and walk to the parking area.

Public transportation: Bus 15 (Mount Tabor) stops at SE 69th Avenue and Yamhill Street. Contact Tri-Met for information about fares and schedules.

Overview: Plympton Kelly, an early settler in this neighborhood, named this hill "Mount Tabor" after he read about a battle fought by the French against the Moslems near Mount Tabor in Palestine. Not until 1912, many years after the hill was developed into a neighborhood park, was it discovered to be an extinct volcano. The summit is 600 feet above the surrounding area.

Paved roads, good views, and many dirt jogging paths make this a popular park with walkers, bicyclists, and runners. Many flights of steps throughout the park help people climb the steep slopes. A reporter for the *Oregonian* once counted 257 steps in all!

The three small pools are actually some of Portland's reservoirs, completed in 1894. Their stonework and castlelike buildings punctuate the park's natural beauty.

The walk

➤Leave the Taylor Street parking lot at the portable toilets and go straight across the main road. The road curves slightly to the left. The roads in this park are unmarked, but as one mother pushing a baby carriage said, "It looks as if you can get lost, but you really can't. All the roads curve back to the starting point."

➤You will come to a wide area where several roads come together. Go straight across this area to the junction of two roads, and then take the road on your right up the hill. This road is steep, but you will see many bicyclists and people pushing strollers up the hill. It is occasionally open to cars. Since it is winding, motorists cannot always see you, so be sure to keep to the left side.

You will come to two sets of stairs. One goes up the hill to your right, and the other goes down the hill to your left. A tennis court lies far below the road on your left. Ferns, wildflowers, and the leathery evergreen bush called salal hug the bank on your right.

➤Pass the stairs and follow the paved road as it curves around to the top of Mount Tabor.

➤Look for the stone steps just beyond the wide area at the crest. Take these up to the statue of Harvey Scott that crowns the grassy summit above the road.

➤Lovely old Douglas-firs crown the summit of Mount Tabor. As you stroll across this knoll, you may notice a City of Portland benchmark in the ground. This is a survey point.

➤After you have finished strolling on the knoll, return to the statue and go down the steps under Scott's hand pointing to the west. There is a small bench here, and you will

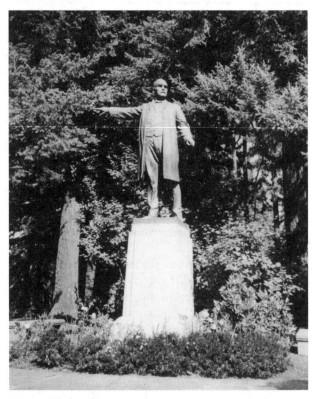

Statue of Harvey Scott.

find others as you proceed to your right on the road around the Harvey Scott Circle.

You will get many glimpses of Portland through gaps in the trees. There is a great view of the city near the north end of the circle. The charming building on the north side of the road that resembles a small French cottage is actually a former restroom building. Vandalism has unfortunately forced its closure.

200

of interest

The Statue and the Sculptor

This statue of Harvey W. Scott, 1838–1910, was made by Gutzon Borglum, who later became famous for carving Mount Rushmore.

Harvey Scott's family came west on the Oregon Trail in 1852, when he was a boy of 14. He later became the first graduate of Pacific University. At age 27, he wrote an editorial on the death of Abraham Lincoln that gained him the editorship of the *Oregonian.* His style was referred to as "conservative and classical." Scott became a "molder of opinion in Oregon and the nation," and one of the movers and shakers of early Portland. He adamantly opposed woman's suffrage, even though his sister, Abigail Scott-Duniway, was one of Oregon's early leaders of the movement.

The sculptor, John Gutzon de la Mothe Borglum, was born in Idaho in 1867. A prolific painter and sculptor, he created 170 public monuments. This larger-than-life statue is relatively small compared to Borglum's other works. He had large-scale visions. Stone Mountain in Georgia is one example of his designs, although other sculptors completed it. Another of Borglum's works, a massive marble head of Abraham Lincoln, is displayed in the rotunda of the Capitol in Washington, D.C. A bronze casting of that head is at Lincoln's tomb in Springfield, Illinois; another is in a public park in Oslo, Norway, and it was also used as a model for the Lincoln profile on Mount Rushmore in the Black Hills of South Dakota. Borglum started the Mount Rushmore project in 1927. It was completed in 1942, eight months after his death.■

➤Proceed around the knoll's north end to the bench inscribed with the words, "Take time to relax and watch the world around you." Diagonally across from this bench are three flights of steps going down the hill. These lead back to the road near the playground. You can take these steps down—they are fairly steep—or continue on the paved road back to the statue to retrace your path down the hill.

➤At the bottom of the hill, continue to the area where the roads meet. You have gone about 1 mile and can easily return to your car from here.

If you wish to see more of the park, go around the barrier and follow the road beyond. This is a favorite area for dog walking, since only park vehicles are allowed on this road, Reservoir Loop Drive.

The road winds downhill. You can hear birdsong over the noise of distant traffic. A soapbox derby track is down the hill on your right, and you can see a large reservoir on the far side of the track. Continue past the trail leading off to the left, and you will see a smaller reservoir on your left.

➤Ignore another trail and a service road going off to the left. Keep on the main road around the hill—known as Poison Oak Hill—until you reach the large reservoir.

➤Follow the road along the tall fence on the west side of this reservoir. Notice the stone buildings that house machinery. You can see the soapbox derby track on the far side of the reservoir, while another reservoir lies down the hill on your left. Ahead are blue gates.

➤Go through these gates, take the road on the right, going uphill. This continuation of Reservoir Loop Drive has two-way vehicular traffic.

➤Continue up this curving road. Walk on the left side of the road and listen carefully, since you cannot always see cars coming down the hill.

➤Pass a gravel trail with steps on your left and two small dirt trails on your right. Stay on the road and continue up "Picnic Hill" until you see the roof of the picnic shelter. A basketball court is down the hill on your left.

Just ahead you will see large lava boulders identifying the location of the volcano. You can read the sign telling about the cinder cone, while viewing the cinders on the hillside across from you.

➤After reading the sign, continue to your right to your starting point in the parking lot.

walk **18**

Convention Center and Lloyd Center

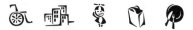

General location: Northeast Portland, just east of Interstate 5.

Special attractions: The Oregon Convention Center, the Rose Garden and Coliseum sports arenas, the Lloyd Center shopping mall, and the trendy Broadway shopping district.

Difficulty rating: Easy, flat, entirely on paved sidewalk with curb cuts.

Distance: 4 miles.

Estimated time: 2 hours.

Services: Wheelchair-accessible restrooms can be found in the Lloyd Center, the Convention Center, and the State Office Building. You will pass many restaurants and stores on this walk.

Restrictions: The Lloyd Center Mall is open weekdays from 10 A.M. to 9 P.M. and Sundays from 11 A.M. to 6 P.M. The Convention Center, Coliseum, and Rose Garden hours vary. Dogs must be leashed and their droppings picked up.

For more information: Contact the Portland Oregon Visitors Association or the Lloyd Center Mall.

Getting started: This walk starts at Lloyd Center at the intersection of Multnomah Street and 9th Avenue. From Interstate 5, take Exit 302A, Convention Center, and turn onto eastbound Weidler Street. Follow the signs to Lloyd Center. At 9th Avenue, turn right and park at Lloyd Center. Parking garages and lots are situated at all four corners of the large mall: Halsey and 9th, Halsey and 15th, Multnomah and 9th, and Multnomah and 15th.

Public transportation: The MAX light-rail runs frequently between Pioneer Place, Lloyd Center, and the Oregon Convention Center. The trains for Lloyd Center leave on the Yamhill Street side of Pioneer Place. The Vintage Trolley Station is by Holladay Park on the Multnomah Street side of Lloyd Center. These trolley replicas have been in use since 1991, traveling between Lloyd Center and Pioneer Place. They operate daily at no charge from March to New Year's Day. Call Tri-Met or the Vintage Trolley for schedules and other information.

Overview: This busy convention and shopping district is easily reached by car, light rail, bus, or trolley. The Oregon Convention Center, the Rose Garden, and the State Office Building are recent developments designed to improve and upgrade the east side of Portland. Many new hotels have been constructed for convention visitors, and many trendy stores and restaurants occupy the old shops and houses along Broadway.

The walk

►Begin this walk at the winning sculpture *Capitalism*, on the Lloyd Center entrance plaza on the southwest corner of the mall, which is between the Nordstrom department store and Stanford's Restaurant on the corner of Multnomah Street and 9th Avenue. The sculpture consists of a classical Ionic capital topped by fifty stacked "coins," each with a funny or serious quotation about money around its edge—a reminder that money is of vital importance to any marketplace. The sculpture is surrounded by a pool.

►Walk past Stanford's on the Multnomah Street side of Lloyd Center. You can see the DoubleTree Portland across the street.

►Pass the Meier and Frank Department Store entrance, and continue to the covered parking lot at the southeast corner of the building. Several other winning art pieces are on display in this lot. Six objects resembling metal mailboxes stand on the concrete curb just inside the lot. These are Christine Bourdette's *Consumer Reliquaries*. Look through the window in each box to view different aspects of the shopping experience. One "Reliquary" contains a glass and aluminum shopping bag by Liz Mapelli.

Free Flow, a bronze sculpture by Al Goldsby, is along the wall at the right end of the parking lot. It is one of the sculptures created for the mall's original opening. At that time, it was a two-tiered waterfall, but it has been redesigned to depict a river to fit this new location.

►Return to Multnomah Street and find the mosaic figure in the sidewalk. Artist Bill Will used a variety of materials in this *Sidewalk Robot*.

►Turn right and retrace your steps to the Meier and Frank entrance.

Convention Center and Lloyd Center

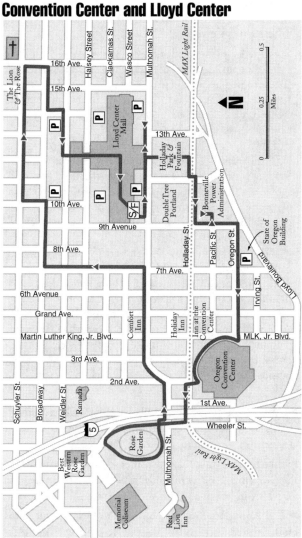

Special thanks to DoubleTree Portland for help with this map.

of interest

The Lloyd Center Mall

Ralph Lloyd dreamed of turning Portland's east side into a vital shopping district, but the Depression and World War II interrupted his plans. He finally opened Lloyd Center in 1960. At the time, it was the first shopping mall in Oregon, the largest urban mall in the United States, and the first to have an ice-skating rink.

Lloyd Center is still growing and expanding, and the mall and rink were recently renovated. The center now contains more than 200 stores and restaurants. The mall sponsors a free Kid's Club with treats, activities, and a club newsletter. The Information Desk is on the lowest level beneath the escalator, and you can find out there about special services and events.

Flight, a sculpture by Portland artist Tom Hardy, was commissioned when the Lloyd Center originally opened. This huge flock of geese now flies above the food court on the third level of the mall. When Lloyd Center was renovated, it sponsored a regional competition for new art to be displayed. Larry Kirkland won the competition with his sculpture, *Capitalism*. This stands outside the center's front entrance; other winning art pieces are also displayed outside.■

➤Cross at the signal into Holladay Park, named after Ben Holladay, a railroad entrepreneur known to many as "a sharpster, a con man, and a rake."

➤Take the sidewalk past the center fountain surrounded by a bed of roses. Go to Holladay Street, where there are stops for MAX light rail and the Vintage Trolley.

➤Turn right onto Holladay and walk to 11th Avenue. Cross Holladay and 11th.

➤Continue straight ahead to 9th Avenue. You can find a drinking fountain on the northeast corner of Holladay and 9th.

➤Turn left onto 9th. The large marble building you are passing is the headquarters of the Bonneville Power Administration. It takes up two entire blocks between Holladay and Lloyd Boulevard.

➤Continue south to the middle of the block, opposite Pacific Street. Turn left onto the walkway between two polished black stone walls.

➤Go toward the building entrance, but turn left before you reach the silver doors. Go toward the outdoor eating area and children's playground.

Across from the eating area and on your left is another of Portland's outdoor sculptures. This large marble wall is divided into ten sections, each punctuated with darker stone. The water flowing over the wall symbolizes Bonneville's association with hydroelectric power.

➤Return on the walkway by which you entered. Go back to 9th.

➤Turn left onto 9th toward Lloyd Boulevard.

➤At the intersection of 9th and Lloyd, turn right and cross at the crosswalk to Oregon Street.

The large circular building ahead of you is a state office building. Glass murals by Hal Bond and Ruth Brockman illustrating legends of Multnomah Falls and the Bridge of the Gods are inside. So is Don Merkt's mixed-media interpretation of the Oregon state motto, "She Flies with Her Own Wings." You will also find public restrooms here.

➤Proceed to 7th Avenue. On the corner of 7th and Oregon is a metered parking lot for visitors. Notice the interesting bronze called *Ideals*. Look inside these classically designed flowing robes and draped hood to see . . . nothing at all.

►Cross 7th Avenue at the crosswalk. The large building straight ahead is the Oregon Convention Center.

►Walk the three blocks to the center. Use the push buttons to operate the traffic signals at Grand Avenue and Martin Luther King Boulevard. Cross Martin Luther King Boulevard into the entrance courtyard of the Convention Center.

►Turn left before you reach the entrance doors, and go to the signpost explaining Portland's water supply system. Just beyond this signpost is *Host Analog*. The creator sawed a large Douglas-fir into pieces and arranged them to resemble a broken Roman column. Then a watering system was installed, seeds and seedlings were planted in the segments, and the column became a typical Oregon "nurse log." The explanatory sign includes pictures showing how the piece looked when it was installed in 1991, and you can see how it has grown and changed in the intervening years.

Bronze wind bells nearby commemorate Oregon's sister relationship with Ulsan, South Korea. More artwork is displayed in the lobby and restrooms of the Convention Center. If the center is closed, you can still see some of it by peering through the glass doors. A dragon boat donated by Portland's sister city, Kaohsiung, Taiwan, hangs in the distance under the green glass tower to the south. This is the same type of boat you might see on the Willamette River when rowers are practicing for competitions during the Rose Festival. Under the green glass tower to the north is a bronze Foucault pendulum that swings over a halo of gilded rays and a blue, inlaid terrazzo floor.

►Walk north around the center toward the Holladay Street entrance. You can see the Holiday Inn and the Best Western

Inn at the Convention Center on the corner of Holladay and Martin Luther King Boulevard.

Two bell circles of different designs create a "sound garden." The wind bells were donated by the Republic of China, and the temple bells were gifts from two of Portland's sister cities: Ulsan, South Korea, and Sapporo, Japan.

➤Cross Holladay at the traffic signal. Follow the walkway across the MAX tracks.

➤Turn left and walk to 1st Avenue.

➤Cross 1st at the signal and go under Interstate 5. The trolley garage is here. A large window displays one of the original Lloyd Center trolley cars.

➤Continue to Wheeler Street and turn right. A sign at this corner of the building tells how Dr. Lawrence Griffith and other volunteers managed to get the rail system and trolley service reactivated.

➤Continue to Multnomah. A sculpture resembling the Statue of Liberty's fallen crown is on the traffic median to your left across the street. This is one of three pieces by Ilan Averbuca representing aspects of Antoine de Saint Exupery's story of *The Little Prince*.

➤Take the crosswalk into the Rose Quarter Plaza. You will walk around the large circular glass Rose Garden, home of the NBA Portland Trail Blazers basketball team.

➤Turn to your left on the walkway. Ahead is a large square with jets of water spraying up and down in a random pattern. This is a favorite play place for kids who do not mind getting wet. The title, *Essential Elements*, seems apropos at night when flames leap up from the two stone columns in the center of the jets of water. The Cucina! Cucina! Restaurant is just beyond the fountain.

➤Turn to your right onto the walkway between the restaurant and the Niketown store. Continue to the main plaza. Memorial Coliseum, home to the Winter Hawks hockey team and the Portland Power women's basketball team, is on your left. This was the former home of the Trail Blazers. Inside the Coliseum are some memorial fountains dedicated to war veterans.

➤Continue along the brick path by the ticket office. You will come to a short street, Winning Way. Across the way is a large bronze wing on a grassy knoll in front of the Best Western Rose Garden Motel. This is another "Little Prince" sculpture. You will not see the third sculpture on this walk.

➤Stay on the south and west side of Winning Way. Walk to the right, past the Rose Garden, to the signal at Multnomah and Wheeler Streets. Turn left. Cross Wheeler at the light.

➤Keep on the left (north) side of Multnomah for four blocks, past the Comfort Inn, to Grand Avenue.

➤Cross Grand. You can see signs for the Lloyd Center. Across the street are three double fountains in front of the Kaiser Permanente Building.

➤Continue straight for two more blocks to 7th Avenue.

➤Cross 7th and turn left. Continue north for five blocks to Broadway. Turn right. Broadway is another up-and-coming shopping area with many good restaurants and interesting stores—a great place to window shop.

➤Continue straight on Broadway for three blocks and then cross 10th Avenue.

➤Turn left onto 10th and go one block to Schuyler Street. Turn right and proceed to 16th Avenue. As you walk along Schuyler, you are passing through the Irvington District. This was the original land claim of William Irving, a

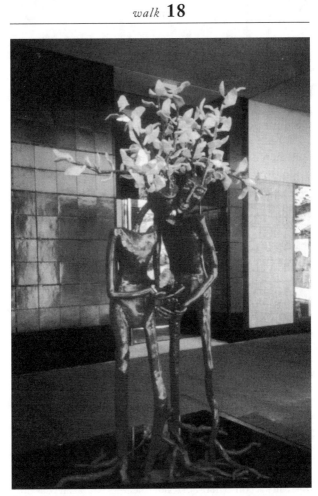

In the Treetops.

seafaring Scotsman. It is a neighborhood in transition. At the corner of Schuyler and 15th Avenue, you can see a lovely old Queen Anne-style home that has been renovated to serve as a bed-and-breakfast, The Lion and the Rose. Other old houses have been torn down or remodeled into apartments. Old trees provide shade over the sidewalks.

When you reach 16th, look across to the stone Presbyterian church on the northeast corner. This is the church attended by Beverly Cleary, author of the children's books that star Ramona Quimby. In one book, Ramona played a sheep in a Christmas pageant at this church.

➤ Turn right and go one block to Broadway.

➤ Cross Broadway, turn right, and go two blocks.

➤ Turn left onto 14th and walk one block to Weidler Street.

➤ Turn right, cross 14th, and proceed back to 12th Avenue. You will pass Holladay Market, a shopping adjunct to Lloyd Center. It contains small restaurants and other interesting spots for browsing.

➤ At 12th Avenue, cross Weidler at the light.

➤ Continue straight down the walkway between J. J. Newberry and a U.S. Bank branch. Margarita Leon's bright red sculpture is impossible to miss. *In the Tree Tops* is a delightful piece featuring two figures with green leaves growing from their heads. In their hands, they cradle a tiny house. This was another winner of the Lloyd art competition.

➤ Cross Halsey Street and enter Lloyd Center. You are on the mall's second (middle) level. The food court can be found on the third level.

➤ Go straight to the center of the mall. Stop at the railing and look down to get a good view of skaters whirling around on the year-round ice rink. Then take the escalator down to the first level.

➤Continue straight ahead toward Nordstrom. The exit to Multnomah and 9th is to the left just before this store. Go through the exit doors, and you will be back at your starting point.

walk 19

Beverly Cleary's Neighborhoods

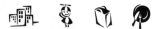

General location: Northeast Portland, about 2 miles east of the Convention Center in the neighborhoods known as Hollywood and Laurelhurst.

Special attractions: If you or your children love Beverly Cleary's children's books, you will all enjoy walking through the Hollywood neighborhood, the setting for many of them. This walk also includes neighboring Laurelhurst, a lovely residential area of early-century homes. You will pass a small lake in Laurelhurst Park.

Difficulty rating: Easy. Entirely on sidewalk. There is one noticeable hill and a ramped climb on the pedestrian walkway over the freeway; otherwise the route is flat.

Distance: 7 miles, but the walk may be divided in two.

Estimated time: 4 hours for the entire 7 miles.

Services: Restaurants can be found in the commercial area around Hancock and 40th Avenue. There are restrooms in Grant Park, at the Hollywood MAX station, and in Laurelhurst Park.

Restrictions: Since these are old neighborhoods, overgrown trees and bushes crowd many sidewalks. Because there are places without curb cuts, the walk is not suitable for wheelchairs. Strollers are fine. No swimming or wading is allowed in the lake in Laurelhurst Park.

For more information: Contact Portland Parks and Recreation or the Multnomah County Library.

Getting started: From Interstate 84 (eastbound), take the 33rd Avenue exit. (Westbound traffic exits at 43rd Avenue.) Turn left (north), and cross Broadway and then Schuyler Street. At Hancock Street turn left into the parking lot for Kienow's grocery store. You may park your car here.

Public transportation: The MAX light-rail stops at the Hollywood Transit Center. You can take Bus 10 (NE 33rd Avenue) from there to the Grant Park playground. If you use the bus, start and finish your walk at the Sculpture Garden just south of the playground. Contact Tri-Met for information about fares and schedules.

Overview: Beverly Cleary has been writing award-winning children's books since the 1950s. Cleary used the Hollywood neighborhood, where she grew up, as the setting for her books about Beezus and Ramona Quimby, Henry Huggins, Ellen Tebbetts, and Otis Spofford. The neighborhood has not changed much. You will walk by Cleary's childhood homes and see some of the schools, parks, and other places that are named in her books. Cleary also set a few scenes in

Beverly Cleary's Neighborhoods

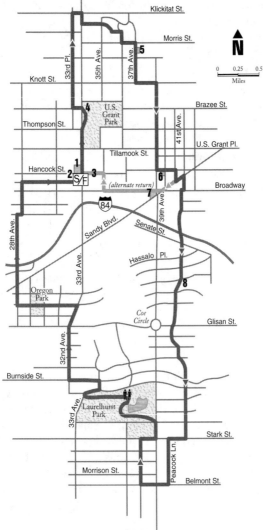

Points of Interest
  1 Fernwood Middle School
  2 Kienow's Grocery Store and Parking Lot
  3 Beverly Cleary's home at 3340 Hancock Street
  4 Beverly Cleary Sculpture Garden
  5 Cleary House at 2924 37th Avenue
  6 Hollywood Branch Library
  7 YMCA
  8 Laurelhurst School

the Laurelhurst neighborhood, which is directly to the south on the other side of the freeway.

The walk takes you past some elegant old homes on streets that curve around a central traffic circle. You will pass the specially designed gates that originally separated the residences from their more mundane surroundings. The developers were influenced by the "City Beautiful" ideas that became popular after the 1893 World's Fair and Columbian Exhibition in Chicago. Developers had already created an upscale Laurelhurst subdivision in Seattle and wanted to establish the same kind of neighborhood in Portland. The Frederick Law Olmsted firm of landscape architects developed the park, and it became known as one of the loveliest on the West Coast.

The walk

➤Begin this walk at Kienow's grocery store at 33rd Avenue and Schuyler Street. Cleary used the store parking lot as the setting for several incidents in her books. In *Ramona the Pest*, Ramona lost her brand-new boots when she got stuck in the mud during the store's construction. She picked burrs here to make a crown for her head in *Ramona and Her Father*, when she got bored waiting for her father to finish meeting with her teacher. This is also where Henry's dog, Ribsy, got a parking ticket in *Henry and Beezus*.

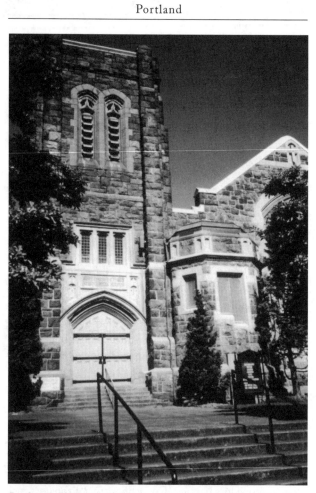

Presbyterian Church on 16th Avenue and Schuyler Street. This is where Ramona was a lamb in the Christmas pageant.

►Exit the parking lot on the Hancock Street side. Across the street to the north is Fernwood Middle School, which was the elementary school Cleary attended as a first grader. Her own first year was miserable, but she compensated for it in *Ramona the Pest* when she created for Ramona the kind of teacher she would have preferred.

►Cross 33rd Avenue at the signal. There is a walk button on the post.

►Walk half a block to 3340 Hancock Street. This is the house in which Cleary lived from fourth grade to sixth grade. The Craftsman-style bungalow is similar to others in the neighborhood, but every house has its own distinguishing touches in doorways, eaves, and windows. This is still a family neighborhood, and it looks much as it did when Cleary was growing up. As you walk, you can imagine Henry, Beezus, and Ramona riding past you on their bikes and jumping rope in the driveways.

►Return to 33rd Avenue and turn right, crossing Hancock. From here you can see the front entrance that was added to Fernwood when it became a middle school.

►Proceed north for two blocks, crossing Tillamook Street and U .S. Grant Place. This was a popular street for drag racers in the 1950s, so it was one of the first in the city to have planters installed in its middle to slow down the traffic.

►You are at the south end of U.S. Grant Park. Continue north on 33rd Avenue along the west side of the park. This is the park in which Henry Huggins dug up night crawlers to sell so that he could reimburse a friend for his lost football.

Note the many examples of English cottages on the other side of 33rd. Shingled roofs designed to imitate thatched roofs make them easily recognizable. Small arched windows under the eaves display tiny balconies suitable for fairy-tale princesses, and the main windows are often trimmed with beautiful beveled glass.

Across the park to your right you can see Cleary's alma mater, U.S. Grant High School. Cleary worked on the school newspaper and wrote a script for a Girls League play. Her teachers chose Cleary to star in the show. The school may look familiar to you because the title character in *Mr. Holland's Opus* was based on a former band teacher at Grant High. The movie was filmed here.

➤Just past the street sign for Thompson Street, take the blacktop walkway on your right into the park; then take the

of interest

The Beverly Cleary Sculpture Garden

This garden was built by the Friends of Henry and Ramona, a volunteer group of teachers, librarians, neighbors, and businesspeople. It was funded by donations from Cleary fans throughout the United States and Canada.

Portland artist Lee Hunt created these life-sized figures of Ribsy, Henry, and Ramona. She used real 1950s clothing on wax models to get the right textures. Ramona, in new boots and flying raincoat, gaily splashes in the fountain. Henry, with a Band-Aid on one hand and an apple bulging from the pocket of his oddly fastened jacket, looks bemused. Ribsy seems surprised at water squirting between his paws. One neighborhood resident claims she's seen dogs try to rub noses with the statue of Ribsy.

Take time to read the titles of Cleary's books etched in the red granite stones surrounding the fountain. Then take a look at the map behind Henry. It uses illustrations by Louis Darling, the original artist, to show where many events in the books take place. ∎

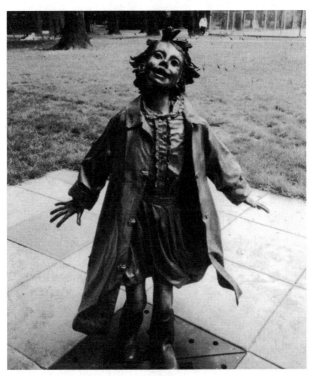

Ramona, Beverly Cleary Sculpture Garden.

first path to your left. The bronze figures ahead of you are part of the Beverly Cleary Sculpture Garden.

➤After you finish studying the map, exit the sculpture garden by the figure of Ribsy and take the path back to the walkway. Turn right, and go down the steps to 33rd Avenue.

➤Cross 33rd at the crosswalk carefully. There are no signals here.

➤Go straight ahead on Brazee Street for one block to 32nd Place.

➤Turn right onto 32nd Place, cross Brazee, and continue north for four blocks to Klickitat Street. Cleary set her books on Hancock Street but preferred the sound of Klickitat.

➤Turn right onto Klickitat and walk up the hill for one block to 33rd Avenue.

➤Look up to your left. You are halfway up the 33rd Avenue Hill. This street used to be closed to traffic when it snowed, and Henry Huggins liked to slide down it on his Flexible Flyer sled.

➤Cross 33rd. Turn right. Go one block to Siskiyou Street, cross and turn left.

➤Cross 34th and 35th Avenues and follow the sidewalk that curves to the right. Take the first left, and you will still be on Siskiyou Street. Continue to 36th Avenue.

➤Turn right at 36th Avenue and go to Morris. Turn left, crossing 36th.

➤Continue one block to 37th and turn right. Cross Morris.

➤Find 2924 37th Avenue. Cleary moved to this tan house with brown trim when she was in sixth grade. She chose the front bedroom for her own, feeling it would put greater distance between her and her parents in their back bedroom. Her father bought her a bike so she could get back and forth to Fernwood School.

Cleary's best friend, Claudine Klum, lived only a block away. Claudine was the inspiration for Ellen's best friend Austine in the book *Ellen Tebbits*, and her house became the model for the Huggins family home.

➤Continue on 37th and cross Stanton to Knott Street.

➤Cross Knott Street and turn left. In the book *Henry*

Huggins, Henry got four kittens at a rummage sale. He was on his way to Knott Street to ask Mr. Capper for a job as a paper boy, and the kittens were hidden in his jacket during the interview.

➤Turn right onto 39th Avenue and continue south to Tillamook Street. The Hollywood shopping district begins at Tillamook Street. You can find small coffee bars and restaurants in this area. Ellen Tebbits, the main character in the book of the same name, lived near Tillamook and 41st Avenue.

➤Continue two more blocks. Cross Hancock. Turn left and cross 39th. Continue one block to the Hollywood branch of the Multnomah County Library. In the 1950s, this new building replaced the Carnegie building that was home to the Rose City Library.

Cleary decided to pursue a career as a writer after winning a $2 first prize in an essay contest. Later, she found out that no one else had entered. Her mother argued that she would need a more reliable way to earn a living. Because the Rose City library was Cleary's favorite refuge, she became a librarian before she began writing stories.

➤From the library, cross 40th Avenue and continue to 41st Avenue.

➤Cross 41st and turn right, passing the Payless Drug Store, the model for the Colossal Drugstore in Cleary's books. In *Otis Spofford*, the Spofford School of Dance is located over this drugstore.

➤Stop at Sandy Boulevard. From here you can see the Hollywood Theater, an exuberant example of Art Deco; it stands on the other side of Sandy between 41st and 42nd Avenues. The theater has recently been restored through community donations. Notice the embellishments on the face of the building. It was considered one of Portland's most

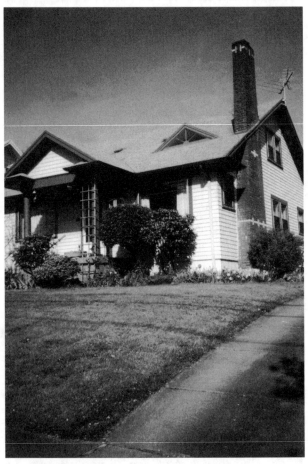

Beverly Cleary's house on NE 37th Avenue.

226

magnificent theaters when it was built in 1926. In the days of silent movies, the organist and the Wurlitzer organ rose slowly from the basement. The theater was so well known that it gave its name to this district, which was originally known as Rose City Park.

(*Author's note:* You have now gone 2 miles. If you wish to return to your starting point, follow the directions below. You then will have walked nearly 3 miles. If you wish to continue for 4 additional miles on the Laurelhurst Loop, follow the directions below for the loop.)

➤To return to your starting point, veer right on Sandy, and go two blocks to Broadway.

➤Turn right onto Broadway, and go west to 38th Avenue. Just south of this corner, at 1630 NE 38th, is the YMCA. Henry and his friend Scooter swam in its indoor pool.

➤Cross 38th and continue on Broadway for three blocks to 35th Avenue.

➤Turn right on 35th. Go one block north to Schuyler Street.

➤Turn left and continue west for two blocks on Schuyler to 33rd Avenue.

➤Turn right on 33rd. The BP gas station across the street on your left is the one where Henry rode up on the grease rack in the car and where Ribsy stole a policeman's lunch.

➤Continue one block to Hancock. Cross 33rd at the signal. Turn left into Kienow's parking lot for the end of this walk.

Laurelhurst Loop

➤ Cross Sandy Boulevard and turn left. Continue for one block to 42nd Avenue.

➤Turn right onto 42nd Avenue, crossing Broadway, Weidler, and Halsey Streets. Look for the pedestrian overpass signs.

➤Take the overpass up and over the freeway and down the other side to Senate Street. You are now in the Laurelhurst neighborhood.

➤Continue south on 42nd Avenue.

➤Cross Hassalo Street at the signal, then cross Hazelfern Place to Laurelhurst Place. Cross 42nd to Laurelhurst School. This school was the inspiration for Cedarhurst School in *Ramona Quimby, Age 8*. Ramona started third grade here with teacher Mrs. Whaley and became friends with "Yard Ape."

➤As you cross Royal Court and continue south to Glisan, you will notice 42nd Avenue has become 41st. Coe Circle, which contains a statue of Joan of Arc, is one block to your right. Like many traffic circles, this one can cause traffic problems. Cross Glisan carefully as you continue south for four more blocks to Burnside.

➤Cross Burnside at the signal and continue for five more blocks to Stark Street. Turn right onto Stark.

➤Continue for about a block until you see the sign for Peacock Lane. Turn left and cross Stark to the right (west) side of Peacock Lane. Continue straight ahead. This unique English-style neighborhood was a forerunner of today's subdivision tracts. R. F. Wassell, the developer, divided his five acres into 33 lots. He saved money by using a similar design for these five- to seven-room houses. The builders were able to buy materials in large quantities and construct several houses at a time. Each house has distinguishing windows and entryways. Wassell also incorporated the best street lighting available at the time. This combination of quality touches and cookie-cutter styles makes Peacock Lane unique. The area is especially noted for its decorations at Christmastime.

➤Peacock Lane ends at Belmont Street. Turn right onto Belmont for one block and cross 39th Avenue.

➤Turn right again when you reach 38th Avenue and take 38th north for four blocks.

➤Cross Stark Street. Turn right onto Stark to the sidewalk along 39th. Turn left on the sidewalk, cross Oak, and enter Laurelhurst Park.

➤Take the path that bends left to the small spring-fed lake with its resident population of turtles, fish, and ducks. It occasionally freezes over and becomes a good place for ice skating. Otis Spofford and Ellen Tebbits skated here in two of Cleary's books.

This is obviously a well-loved park where people jog, stroll, and walk dogs. Tall, old trees shade benches and picnic tables. Volunteers maintain all park flower beds. There are a horseshoe pit, playgrounds, and courts for tennis, volleyball, and basketball.

➤Walk to the left around the west end of the pond, and then take the asphalt path on your left toward the restrooms. Continue to your left, past picnic areas, to the northwest corner of the park. Exit the park at 33rd Avenue.

➤Turn right to Ankeny and continue past the park until you see the sign for Floral Place. You will find large homes here. Notice the one across the way at number 3316. It could have belonged to a friend of the Great Gatsby in the Roaring Twenties.

➤Turn left and cross Ankeny, keeping on the left side of Floral Place.

➤Continue straight for one block to Burnside.

➤Turn left onto Burnside Street and walk to 32nd Avenue (a continuation of 33rd Avenue). Notice the Laurelhurst gate at this intersection. These gates were designed to separate residential Laurelhurst from the surrounding commercial district.

➤Cross Burnside at the signal.

➤Stay on 32nd to Glisan Street, where you can see another Laurelhurst gate.

➤Look for the push buttons that control the signals. Cross Glisan and 32nd with the lights. On your left is the Greek Orthodox Church of the Holy Trinity.

➤Continue past this church, cross Hoyt Street, and continue one block to Irving Street.

➤Turn left (west) onto Irving for two blocks. When you cross 30th, you will find yourself in Oregon Park. This small neighborhood park is a nice place for children to play.

➤Continue straight through the park. Exit on Irving Street and continue one more block to 28th.

➤Turn right onto 28th and walk two blocks to Sandy Boulevard.

➤Cross Sandy at the walk signal—there is a push button— and continue north to Holladay. The bridge over the freeway is straight ahead. Cleary lived on Halsey Street next to Sullivan's Gulch, the name for the canyon where the freeway is today. Ben Holladay used this gulch for Oregon's first railroad.

➤Cross the freeway and continue straight on the wide sidewalk.

➤Keep heading north. After you cross Wasco Street, you can see the new Hollywood West Fred Meyer store on the right. There are restrooms and a deli inside the store.

➤Cross Clackamas. The sidewalk jogs to the right at Halsey Street. A nice little park is here at the end of the Fred Meyer parking lot; the Hollywood Neighborhood Association negotiated with the store to create the park.

➤Keep on 28th as it jogs left. Cross Weidler. The neighborhood association also arranged for Weidler and other streets to be closed to traffic to keep them from being used as thoroughfares.

➤Cross Broadway. Go straight to Schuyler and turn right.

➤Continue (east) for two blocks. You can see a BP gas station across the street in the third block.

➤Just before you reach 33rd Avenue, cross Schuyler and turn left into Kienow's parking lot. This is the end of this walk.

walk 20

The Grotto

General location: The Grotto is in Northeast Portland, 3 miles south of Portland International Airport.

Special attractions: Gardens, statuary (including a replica of Michelangelo's *Pietá*, chapels, gift shop, and a spectacular view north across the Columbia River.

Difficulty rating: Easy walk on paved paths, with an elevator to the upper gardens.

Distance: 1 mile, including walks on both levels.

Estimated time: 1 hour.

Services: A coffee bar, gift shop, and wheelchair-accessible restrooms are available at the Welcome Center.

Restrictions: A $2 token must be purchased at the Welcome Center or the Visitor Complex to gain access to the upper level of gardens. The Grotto is open daily except on Thanksgiving and Christmas. No pets are permitted.

For more information: Contact the Grotto.

Getting started: From Interstate 205 northbound, take the Sandy Boulevard West exit to NE 85th Avenue. Follow the signs to the Grotto entrance.

Public transportation: Bus 12 (Sandy) stops at the entrance to the Grotto. Contact Tri-Met for information about fares and schedules.

Overview: Only five minutes from Portland International Airport, this 62-acre Roman Catholic sanctuary is a peaceful retreat from the hurry of modern life. Stroll leisurely through the woodsy plaza level, where vines and shrubs muffle the noise of nearby Sandy Boulevard, and admire the replica of Michelangelo's *Pietá* inside a rock grotto. An elevator lifts you to the top of a 110-foot cliff. At the top, you'll find beautifully manicured gardens and incredible views. Statues are everywhere; many of them were carved in Italy from Carrara marble. The Welcome Center contains a gift shop and coffee bar, and the Visitor Complex displays and sells Nativity sets from all over the world. Special religious and musical events often take place on these grounds, and a December "Christmas Festival of Lights" is an outstanding annual event.

The walk

►The walk begins at the parking lot at Sandy Boulevard and 85th Avenue. A large bas-relief sculpture of President John F. Kennedy is to the right of the entrance, a gift from various Catholic organizations.

The Grotto

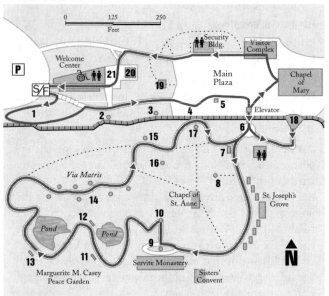

Special thanks to The Grotto for help with this map.

Points of Interest

1 Stations of the Cross
2 Sacred Heart statue
3 St. Philip Benizi statue
4 Grotto Cave, altar, and *Pietà*
5 St. Peregrine mosaic
6 Meyer Memorial Garden Plaza
7 Statue of Our Sorrowful Mother
8 St. Francis of Assisi statue
9 Lithuanian wayside shrine
10 The Seven Sorrows of Mary
11 Glorious Mysteries
12 Sorrowful Mysteries
13 Joyful Mysteries
14 Peace Pole
15 Assumption of Mary statue and rose garden
16 St. Jude Thaddeus statue
17 Directory
18 Marilyn Moyer Meditation Chapel
19 Christus Statue
20 Madonna of Orvieto
21 Clotilde Merlo Plaza

➤Go to the glass-fronted building at the end of the parking area. This is the Welcome Center. Pick up a free map and purchase a token for $2 if you wish to go to the Upper Gardens. Access to these is only by elevator.

➤Leave the Welcome Center and stop to look at the large display case outside. This provides information about the Grotto and what you can see here.

➤Cross the walkway and follow the signs pointing to the Stations of the Cross.

The path winds through a green, quiet area among lovely rhododendrons and tall firs. Fourteen bronze plaques, with figures carved in relief, illustrate highlights of the journey of Jesus to his crucifixion. The first six stations are located on your left.

➤At Station 7, the path turns left and goes slightly uphill. It levels out at Station 8. From here, the station markers will be found on your right.

➤Continue on the path until you reach Station 14, which brings you to steps leading back to the Welcome Center. Bypass these steps, take the path to the right instead, and pass the *Sacred Heart* statue.

➤The next statue is of a kneeling figure with a papal crown on the ground next to him. The statue is of Saint Philip Benizi, a Servite who hid from those who would have elected him pope. The statue is just before the entrance into the Grotto plaza.

Racks of votive candles flank the altar in front of the Grotto Cave, while the recorded sound of Gregorian chants floats through the area. Mass is celebrated in this plaza every Sunday at noon during the summer months.

of interest

The Grotto

When Ambrose Mayer was a small boy in Canada, he prayed for his mother's recovery from a difficult childbirth and promised he would one day do a great work for the Catholic Church. His mother recovered, and Ambrose kept his promise. He became a member of the Order of Servants of Mary (Servites), which had been founded and dedicated to Mary, Mother of Sorrows, in 1233. The order eventually sent him to Portland.

Father Mayer was able to purchase acreage from the Union Pacific Railroad for $3,000 to found this Sanctuary of Our Sorrowful Mother. It was dedicated in 1924, and a cave was carved out of the 110-foot basalt cliff shortly thereafter. The stone from the cliff was used to construct the large altar in front of the Grotto, and a replica of Michelangelo's *Pietà* was installed. The spot became a national sanctuary in 1983, and it has provided a peaceful haven to visitors of all faiths from all over the world ever since.■

➤At the left edge of the altar area is a mosaic icon of Saint Peregrine Laziosi, the patron saint of those suffering from cancer, AIDS, or other life-threatening diseases. The leg sores of this thirteenth-century Servite brother were miraculously cured through prayer the night before his leg was to be amputated.

➤South of the Grotto plaza, against the cliff, is a tall concrete structure housing the elevator. Take the path leading to it, drop your token in the turnstile, and enter the elevator.

➤After the ascent, the elevator doors open onto the Meyer Memorial Garden Plaza. Restrooms can be found to your left. Signs pointing to the Upper Gardens are directly in front of you.

➤Enter the main gardens. On your right, you will see a directory and map. Note the many small pathways leading to various statues and shrines. If you explore any of these, return to the main walkway after your visit.

➤Take the walkway to your left. This passes a small path on the right that leads to the statue of Saint Jude Thaddeus.

➤The main walk goes by large trees marking Saint Joseph's Grove. The statue of Saint Joseph is surrounded by bas-relief panels depicting the joys and sorrows of his life.

The next path to your right leads to the Chapel of Saint Anne. This little chapel is in a lovely garden.

➤Continue on the main walkway, past the Servite Monastery that houses the priests and brothers who staff the Grotto. This building and the sisters' convent in the rear are not open to the public.

In front of the monastery is the statue of the Assumption of Mary, surrounded by a rose garden. The rose bushes were donated by the Royal Rosarians, a group of active civic leaders and sponsors of Portland's annual Rose Festival. The plaque at the base of the fountain honors the group's deceased members.

➤Follow the walkway to the right. Here is the Peace Pole, dedicated in 1988 to prayer for world peace. Each of the four sides bears the message "May peace prevail on earth" inscribed in either English, Japanese, Russian, or Spanish.

➤Continue past a reflection pond to the Marguerite M. Casey Peace Garden, where you will find three sets of plaques by Oregon artist Mary Lewis. These depict the Joyful, Sorrowful, and Glorious mysteries of the Rosary.

Follow the walkway along a small rivulet that leads to a second tranquil pond. The sound and sight of waterfalls and flowing water enhance the serene garden setting.

➤The walkway continues through shady groves along the Via Matris, The Way of Our Sorrowful Mother. Life-sized figures made of white pine are encased in glass housings and surrounded by shrubs. These represent the Seven Sorrows of Mary and were carved prior to 1930 in the Heider Studio of Pietralba, Italy. Originally tinted in pastel colors, they were stripped down to the original wood in 1986.

➤After viewing the last station, where Mary lays her Son in the tomb, a path goes to the right to the Chapel of Saint Anne.

➤Stay on the main walkway to see an ancient Lithuanian wayside shrine on your left. This gift from Portland and Chicago Lithuanians combines the pagan symbols of tree worship with those symbolizing Christianity.

➤Beyond this shrine is a bronze statue of Saint Francis of Assisi with a group of animals; it was created by local artist Michael Florian Denté and dedicated in 1993.

➤Ahead, high on a stone pillar, is the statue of Our Sorrowful Mother, a gift of the Catholic Daughters of the Americas. Walk to the north side and look up to see Mary, shown in that awful moment when she stood at the foot of the Cross and heard Jesus tell John to "Behold thy mother."

➤Cross to the green iron fence to see a magnificent vista of the mountains and Columbia River. You can see Mount St. Helens, Mount Adams, and even Mount Rainier from this viewpoint near the cliff's edge.

➤Return to the walkway that leads you once again into the Meyer Memorial Garden Plaza. Instead of taking the elevator down, cross the plaza and take the walkway leading to the Marilyn Moyer Meditation Chapel. A raised walkway between flowing waterways takes you into the chapel. You will be struck immediately by the stunning view through the beveled-glass bow window, which was once featured in *Architecture* magazine. This window is a work of art and offers one of the best 180-degree views in the Portland area.

Centered in front of this window is a realistic, life-sized wax sculpture entitled *Mother and Child*. This resin and fiberglass piece by John De Andrea was installed here in May 1997. The simply furnished chapel provides a perfect setting for an inspiring view of land and sky as well as for your own meditations.

➤Return to the elevator and descend to the lower level. After you exit, turn right to visit the Chapel of Mary on the east side of the Main Plaza. Daily Mass is celebrated in this beautiful marble sanctuary. Soft light filters in from the 25-foot-high stained-glass window celebrating Christ's Resurrection. Spanish-born José De Soto, an artist who painted movie sets for Fox Studios, created the murals on the chapel walls.

➤As you leave the chapel, turn right and walk to the back of the plaza. Stop in at the Visitor Center, which is staffed with knowledgeable volunteers who can answer almost any question you may have about the Grotto. The gift shop contains a small display of art and an exceptionally large collection of Nativity sets. Created in a wide variety of media reflecting the country of origin, these range from one to twelve inches high and are available for purchase.

➤Leave the Visitor Center, turn right, and pass the Security Center. Restrooms are located in the lower level of this building.

➤Turn left and skirt the west side of the plaza, following the signs to the Christus statue. This bronze statue of Christ carrying His cross to Calvary is set in its own small courtyard within a rhododendron grove.

➤Turn onto the path on your right, following it back to the main walkway.

➤Turn left onto this walkway and go to Clotilde Merlo Plaza. The revolving "Madonna of Orvieto" diorama is on the east side of this plaza. The Welcome Center is on the west side.

➤Take the walkway by the Welcome Center back to your starting point in the parking lot.

walk 21

Airport Way

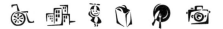

General location: Just east of Interstate 205 and Portland International Airport.

Special attractions: A chance to stretch your legs and enjoy a bit of nature in the midst of the airport-motel district.

Difficulty rating: Easy, flat, entirely on sidewalks with curb cuts.

Distance: 1.5 miles.

Estimated time: 45 minutes.

Services: There are restaurants, restrooms, and water at the motels.

Restrictions: Walk during daylight hours. Glen Widing Drive is well lit, but the bike trail to Marine Drive is not.

For more information: Ask at the reception desks of any of the motels on Airport Way, including the Marriott Courtyard,

Airport Way

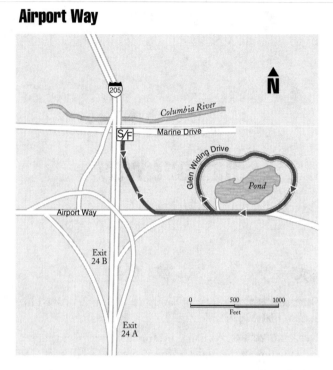

Fairfield Inn, Holiday Inn Express, Shilo Inn, Silver Cloud Inn, and Super 8 Motel.

Getting started: Take Airport Way east underneath Interstate 205 to the junction with Glen Widing Drive. You will see motels on both sides of the strip.

Public transportation: Bus 12 (Sandy) stops on 82nd near the Marriott Courtyard and at the airport. Contact Tri-Met for information about fares and schedules.

242

If you have a long layover between flights, it is possible to take this walk by taking a shuttle bus to one of the motels. Construction at the airport means that pickup stops can change, so check with the guides at the airport and follow signs to the designated area for buses and shuttles.

Overview: This area recently has become a motel and commercial district serving the Portland International Airport. A small pond still remains in the center of the area; it is part of the Columbia River Slough, which the Port of Portland is maintaining as open space, even as development goes on all around it. These slough areas are important watersheds, providing homes to many types of wildlife, as well as a pleasant respite from the bustle of the airport and motels.

The walk

➤ Begin this walk from any of the motels on Airport Way.

➤ Start on the north side of Airport Way. Take the concrete sidewalk west along Airport Way toward Interstate 205. You will see a small pond, part of the Columbia River Slough. This is a natural pond, bordered by brush, willows, and evergreens. As you go by, you may see a great blue heron fishing for dinner. The great blue heron has been Portland's official city bird since 1987.

➤ A concrete bikeway will branch to your right, paralleling the freeway.

➤ Turn right and take the bikeway, following the sign pointing to Marine Drive. The bikeway ends at NE Marine Drive, a well-traveled and busy road. You can see the Columbia River on the other side. A walking path is planned for the future, but at present only bicyclists can safely travel this part of Marine Drive.

➤Look east for a magnificent view of Mount Hood and then retrace your steps to the junction with Glen Widing Drive and Airport Way.

➤Turn left and follow Glen Widing Drive around the pond. You should still have a great view of Mount Hood. Look across a small meadow on your right for another view of the pond. A little farther east, still on your right, is an old Northwest-style home. This style of home was designed to blend into the natural landscape, and at one time it must have fit perfectly into a remote setting overlooking the pond.

➤Continue past the private driveway.

➤Pass the drive into the Fairfield Inn, and you will come once again to Airport Way.

➤Return to your motel.

walk 22

Alderwood Road

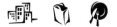

General location: Just west of Interstate 205 and south of Portland International Airport.

Special attractions: This walk offers you a chance to escape from the airport hustle. You walk through a public golf course and can see some of the Columbia River Slough.

Difficulty rating: Easy and flat.

Distance: 1.5 miles.

Estimated time: 45 minutes.

Services: Restaurants and motels.

Restrictions: Alderwood Road lacks shoulders where it crosses the golf course. Traffic also moves slowly in this area. This walk is best undertaken during the day, since there are few lights at night.

Alderwood Road

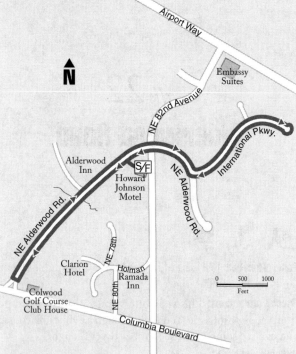

Special thanks to the Port of Portland for help with this map.

For more information: Stop at the reception desks at the Howard Johnson Motel, Alderwood Inn, Clarion Hotel, Embassy Suites Hotel, or Ramada Inn.

Getting started: This walk starts at the Howard Johnson Motel, at the junction of Alderwood Road and NE 82nd Avenue. Take Airport Way east to 82nd Avenue, turn right, and go south. Cross Alderwood Road. The main entrance of the motel is immediately south of this junction. The

Embassy Suites Hotel is at the southeast corner of Airport Way and 82nd Avenue. The Alderwood Inn, Clarion Hotel, and Ramada Inn are nearby.

Public transportation: Bus 12 (Sandy) stops at 82nd and Alderwood, at the Howard Johnson Motel, and at the airport.

If you have a long layover between flights, it is possible to take this walk by taking a shuttle bus to one of the motels. Construction at the airport means that pickup stops can change, so check with the guides at the airport and follow signs to the designated area for buses and shuttles.

Overview: This walk goes through the Portland International Center, a planned business park with a natural environment and campus atmosphere. The Port of Portland is maintaining this part of the Columbia River Slough as open space within developed areas. The slough contains sluggish streams and small ponds and is one of Portland's important watersheds. Home to many forms of wildlife, it makes a pleasant contrast to the busy surroundings.

The walk

➤This walk begins at the parking lot on the north side of the Howard Johnson Motel. Turn left and go to the rear of the motel by buildings C and D. You are now on Alderwood Road.

➤Walk left (south) toward the Alderwood Inn. Golf greens flank the road.

➤Stop at the signal and then cross Cornfoot Road. Alderwood Road continues through the center of the Colwood Golf Course. Privately owned, Colwood is open to the public. The course is frequently rented for tournaments, so walk only on the edges of the course.

➤Look for the sign that says "The ladies tee is across the bridge." Just before the sign, take the path on your left into the golf course. Turn right on the footpath and follow this around to the small footbridge. You are crossing one of the streams of the Columbia River Slough. Look down to see if you can spot any ducks or turtles.

➤On the other side of the bridge, take the path to the right and return to Alderwood Road. This road continues south for another third of a mile and then ends at Columbia Boulevard. The clubhouse for the Colwood Golf Course is just east of this junction. It serves meals throughout the day.

➤Turn around at Columbia Boulevard. Return via the same route to the Howard Johnson Motel.

➤Continue past the back entrance of the motel and on to the junction of 82nd Avenue.

➤Cross 82nd at the signal and continue on Alderwood Road. This area of the airport district is devoted to offices. Concrete sidewalks and manicured green parkways edge the building sites.

➤Continue to International Parkway, which will enter Alderwood Road from the left. Turn left and take International Parkway to the cul-de-sac at the end.

Natural meadows and sloughs surround these new office buildings and road. Overall plans call for these natural areas to become part of the 40-Mile Loop system, which will eventually link all Portland parks in one 140-mile loop.

➤Go around the cul-de-sac and return the way you came.

➤At the junction of International Parkway and Alderwood, cross Alderwood, turn right, cross 82nd at the light, and return to the Howard Johnson Motel.

Appendix A: Other Sights

You may enjoy several other attractions in Portland or nearby. They may not involve much walking, but they have been enjoyed by visitors and Oregonians of all ages.

Hiking

The Columbia Gorge begins in Troutdale, 12 miles east of Portland. It has wonderful waterfalls, gorgeous views, and hiking trails suited to all abilities. Take Interstate 84 eastbound to Exit 35 to access the old Columbia Gorge Scenic Highway. This route passes Vista House at Crown Point, which offers an unusual and spectacular view of the Columbia River along with tourist information and gifts. It continues on to Multnomah Falls where you will have a beautiful view of the falls. The lodge has a dining room, snack bar, and a gift store. The trail to the falls was temporarily closed in the spring of 1998. Ask in the lodge for information about the trail's reopening, as well as information about other nearby trails.

Museums

End of the Trail Interpretive Center. 1726 Washington Street, Oregon City, OR 97405, 503-657-9336. Oregon City is the official end of the Oregon Trail, and the center sits on Abernathy Green, which was the main arrival area for emigrants. The three covered wagon-shaped buildings house live history presentations, a mixed-media show about the journey, exhibits, and a museum store featuring Northwest crafts and heritage items. Call for information about fees, times, and ticket information, or visit the web site at http://www.teleport.com/~eotic.

Oregon Museum of Science and Industry (OMSI).
1945 SE Water Street, Portland (on the east side of the
river, across from the Portland Oregon Visitors Association
Center), 503-797-4000, http://www.omsi.edu. Six exhibit
halls offer hands-on exhibits, live demonstrations, a plan-
etarium, an OMNIMAX theater, and the USS *Blueback* sub-
marine used in the film *Hunt for Red October*. There is a
small restaurant and a gift store.

Portland Children's Museum. 3037 SW Second
Avenue, Portland 97201, 503-823-2227. This museum is
designed for children from six months to ten years old. It
contains exhibits and lots of hands-on activities, such as a
medical center, grocery store, and clay studio.

Appendix B: Contact Information

Throughout this book we have advised you to contact local attractions, museums, and shops to confirm opening times, locations, and entrance fees. The list below gives you the phone numbers and addresses of all the places we mentioned.

Note: The area code for all of Portland is 503.

Oregon Convention Center
777 NE Martin Luther King Jr. Boulevard
PO Box 12210
Portland 97232
235-7575
1-800-791-2250

Pioneer Courthouse Square Association
Pioneer Courthouse Square
701 SW 6th Avenue
Portland 97204
223-1613

Portland Oregon Visitors Association
26 SW Salmon Street
Portland 97204
222-2223
http://www.pova.com
The Portland Oregon Visitors Association has a wealth of information about Portland. If you are in town, stop by the Visitor Center or call them with your questions.

Activities, Attractions, and Museums

Blitz-Weinhard Brewery
1113 W Burnside Street
Portland 97209
223-4351

The Grotto
PO Box 20008
Portland 97220
254-7371

Oregon History Center
1200 SW Park Avenue
Portland 97205
222-1741
http://www.ohs.org

Oregon Maritime Museum
113 SW Naito Parkway
Portland 97204
224-7724
http://www.teleport.com/~omcm/

Oregon Museum of Science and Industry (OMSI)
1945 SE Water Avenue
Portland 97214-3354
797-4000 or 797-OMSI
http://www.omsi.edu/

Portland Center for the Performing Arts
1111 SW Broadway
Portland 97205
448-4305

Portland Police Museum
1111 SW 2nd Street
Portland
823-0019

State of Oregon Sports Hall of Fame
321 SW Salmon Street
Portland 97204
227-7466

World Forestry Center
4033 SW Canyon Road
Portland 97221
228-1367

Parks, Gardens, and Golf Courses

Colwood Golf Club
7213 NE Columbia Boulevard
Portland 97220
254-5515

Eastmoreland Golf Club
2425 SE Bybee Road
Portland 97202
775-2900

The Friends of Crystal Springs Rhododendron Garden
PO Box 86424
Portland 97286

The Friends of Johnson Creek
11820 SE Foster Place
Portland 97266

The Friends of Marquam Nature Park
1041 SW Westwood Court
Portland 97202

The Friends of Powell Butte Nature Park
1038 SE 244th
Gresham 97236

Hoyt Arboretum
4000 SW Fairview Boulevard
Portland 97221
228-8733

Japanese Gardens
611 SW Kingston Avenue
PO Box 3847
Portland 97208
223-1321

Portland Audubon Society and Nature Store
15151 NW Cornell Road
Portland 97210
292-9453

Portland Parks and Recreation
1120 SW Fifth, Suite 1302
Portland 97204
823-2223 V/TT
http://www.parks.ci.portland.or.us

Tryon Creek State Park
11321 SW Terwilliger Boulevard
Portland 97219

Washington Park Zoo
4001 SW Canyon Road
Portland 97221
226-1561

Airport Hotels

Alderwood Inn
7025 NE Airport Road
Portland 97218
255-2700
1-888-987-2700

Clarion Hotel Airport
6233 NE 78th Court
Portland 97218
251-2000
1-800-994-7878

254

Fairfield Inn
11929 NE Airport Way
Portland 97220
253-1400
1-800-228-2800

Holiday Inn Express—Portland Airport
11938 NE Airport Way
Portland 97220
251-9991
1-800-HOLIDAY

Howard Johnson's Airport Hotel
7101 NE 82nd Avenue
Portland 97220
255-6722

Marriott Courtyard
11550 NE Airport Way
Portland 97220-1070
252-3200
1-800-321-2211

Ramada Inn
6221 NE 82nd Avenue
Portland 97220-1302
255-6511
1-800-272-6232

Shilo Suites Hotel
11600 SW Corby Drive
Portland 97225
641-6565, ext. 43

Silver Cloud Inn
11518 NE Glen Widing Drive
Portland 97220
252-2222
1-800-205-7892

Super 8 Motel
11011 NE Holman Street
Portland 97220
257-8988

Convention Center and Lloyd Center Hotels

Best Western Inn at the Convention Center
420 NE Holladay
Portland 97232
233-6331

Best Western Rose Garden Hotel
10 N Weidler Street
Portland 97227-1830
287-9900

Comfort Inn at the Convention Center
431 NE Multnomah Street
Portland 97232-2010
233-7933
1-800-228-5150

DoubleTree Portland—Lloyd Center
1000 NE Multnomah Street
Portland 97232-2111
281-6111

Holiday Inn—Portland Downtown
1021 Grand Avenue
Portland 97232
235-2100
1-800-343-1822

The Lion and the Rose Victorian Bed and Breakfast
1810 NE 15th
Portland 97212
1-800-955-1647
lionrose@ix.netcom.com

Ramada Plaza Hotel
1441 NE 2nd Avenue
Portland 97232
233-2401

Red Lion Portland Inn
1225 N Thunderbird Way
Portland 97227-1822
235-8311
1-800-547-8010

Rodeway Inn—Convention Center
1506 NE 2nd
Portland 97232
231-7665
1-800-228-2000

Downtown Hotels

5th Avenue Suites Hotel
506 SW Washington Street
Portland 97204-1550
222-0001
1-800-711-2971

The Benson Hotel
309 SW Broadway
Portland 97205-3725
228-2000

Days Inn City Center
1414 SW 6th Avenue
Portland 97201-3497
221-1611
1-800-899-0248

DoubleTree Portland—Downtown
310 SW Lincoln Street
Portland 97201-5007
221-0450
1-800-733-5466

Embassy Suites at the Multnomah Hotel
319 SW Pine Street
Portland 97204-2726
279-9000
1-800-EMBASSY

The Governor Hotel
611 SW 10th
Portland 97205-2725
224-3400
1-800-826-1431

The Heathman Hotel
1001 SW Broadway
Portland 97205-3096
241-4100
1-800-551-0011

Hotel Vintage Plaza
422 SW Broadway
Portland 97205-3595
228-1212
1-800-243-0555

Imperial Hotel
400 SW Broadway
Portland 97205-3579
228-7221
1-800-452-2323

Mallory Hotel
729 SW 15th Avenue
Portland 97205-1994
223-6311
1-800-228-8657

The Mark Spencer Hotel
409 SW 11th Avenue
Portland 97205-2633
224-3293
1-800-548-3934

Marriott Hotel—Downtown Portland
1401 SW Naito Parkway
Portland 97201-5192
226-7600
1-800-228-9290

The Portland Hilton Hotel
921 SW 6th Avenue
Portland 97204-1202
226-1611
1-800-HILTONS

RiverPlace Hotel
1510 SW Harbor Way
Portland 97201-5169
228-3233

The Riverside
50 SW Morrison Street
Portland 97204-3390
221-0711
1-800-899-0247

Schools

Lewis and Clark College
0615 SW Palatine Hill Road
Portland 97219-7879
244-6161
http://www.lclark.edu

Portland State University
724 SW Harrison
Portland 97207
725-3000
http://www.pdx.edu

Reed College
3203 SE Woodstock Boulevard
Portland 97202
771-1112
1-800-547-4750
http://www.reed.edu

Shopping

Lloyd Center
2201 Lloyd Center (corner of NE 9th and Multnomah)
Portland 97232
282-2511

Powell's City of Books
1005 W. Burnside
Portland 97209
228-4651
1-800-878-7323
http://www.powells.com

Transportation

Tri-Met Transportation District of Oregon

1412 SE 17th Avenue
Portland 97202
238-RIDE
TTY 238-5811
http://www.tri-met.org

All buses and light rail transportation services are part of the Tri-Met system.

The Vintage Trolley

323-7363

Also part of Tri-Met, the free trolley runs between the Lloyd Center and Pioneer Courthouse Square every half hour from 10 A.M. to 3 P.M. on weekdays, 10 A.M. to 6 P.M. every weekend.

Appendix C: Great Tastes

As you walk through Portland, you will notice many small coffee and/or sandwich shops, pubs, and other types of eateries. They can be found along the streets, on the college campuses, and inside the shopping centers.

There are far too many to list in this guide. The *Official Visitors Guide* available at the Portland Oregon Visitors Association lists restaurants by type of food and price. *Independent Living Resources* has a guide to local restaurants that are wheelchair accessible. Write to them at 4506 SE Belmont Street, Portland 97215 or call 232-7411 for information.

The following list is of some of the major restaurants that you will pass while doing walks listed in this book. The starred restaurants are wheelchair accessible.

Atwater's Restaurant and Bar*
111 SW 5th Avenue, 30th Floor
Portland 97204
275-3600

B. Moloch/The Heathman Bakery and Pub*
901 SW Salmon Street
Portland 97205
227-5700

Carnival Restaurant
2805 SW Sam Jackson Park Road
Portland 97201
227-4244

Couch Street Fish House
105 NW 3rd Avenue
Portland 97209
223-6173

Cucina! Cucina! Italian Café
One Center Court, Suite 130
Portland 97232
238-9800

Dan and Louis Oyster Bar Restaurant and Museum
208 SW Ankeny Street
Portland 97204
227-5906

Esplanade Restaurant at RiverPlace
1510 Harbor Way
Portland 97201
228-3233

Great China Seafood Restaurant
336 NW Davis
Portland 97205
228-2288

House of Louie*
331 NW Davis
Portland 97205
228-9898

Jake's Famous Crawfish
401 SW 12th Avenue
Portland 97205
226-1419

Jake's Grill at the Governor Hotel
611 SW 10th Avenue
Portland 97205
220-1850

Riverside Café and Bar
50 SW Morrison Street
Portland 97204
221-0711
1-800-899-0247

Saigon Kitchen
835 NE Broadway
Portland 97232
281-3669

Stanford's Restaurant at Lloyd Center
913 Lloyd Center (NE corner of 9th and Multnomah)
Portland 97232
335-0811

Zefiro*
500 NW 21st Avenue
Portland 97209
226-3394

Appendix D: Useful Phone Numbers

Note: The front of the US DEX Yellow Pages contains many toll-free numbers for information on almost anything you can imagine.

Multnomah County Library
248-5123
http://www.multnomah.lib.or.us

Poison Control
494-8968

Portland Fire Bureau
Emergency: 911
Non-emergency: 823-3700

Portland Police Bureau
Emergency: 911
Non-emergency: 230-2121

Time and Temperature
243-7575

Hospitals

Department of Veterans Affairs Medical Center
220-8262

Eastmoreland Hospital
Southeast Portland
2900 SE Steele
234-0411

Legacy Emanuel Hospital
Northeast Portland
2801 N. Gantenbein
413-2200

Legacy Good Samaritan Hospital and Medical Center
Northwest Portland
1015 NW 22nd
413-7711

Oregon Health Sciences University (OHSU)
Southwest Portland
3181 SW Sam Jackson Park Road
494-8311

Providence Portland Medical Center
Northeast Portland
4805 NE Glisan Street
215-1111

Providence Milwaukie Medical Center
Southeast Portland
10150 SE 32nd Avenue
Milwaukee, OR 97222

Providence St. Vincent Medical Center
Southwest Portland
9205 SW Barnes Road
Portland 97225
216-1234

Newspapers

Oregonian
221-8240
http://www.oregonlive.com

Portland Parent
638-1049
http://www.portlandparent.com

Willamette Week
243-2122
http://www.wweek.com

Appendix E: Read All About It

Want to learn more about Portland? The following books are but a sample of the many you might enjoy.

Fiction

Beverly Cleary has written many children's books set in Portland and two autobiographies about her growing up. She gives a good view of everyday life in the city. Her two autobiographies are *A Girl from Yamhill*, New York: Morrow, 1988, and *My Own Two Feet*, New York: Morrow, 1996.

Multnomah County Library sponsors a web page with lots of Cleary information at http://www.multnomah.lib.or.us/lib/kids/cleary.html. Cleary's Portland children's books were all published by Morrow between 1950 and 1981:

Henry Huggins
Henry and Beezus
Henry and the Clubhouse
Henry and the Paper Route
Henry and Ribsy
Ribsy
Ellen Tebbits
Otis Spofford
Beezus and Ramona
Ramona the Pest
Ramona the Brave
Ramona and Her Father
Ramona and Her Mother
Ramona Quimby, Age 8
Ramona Forever

Haycox, Ernest. *The Long Storm.* Boston: Little, Brown and Company, 1946

Portland author Ernest Haycox's *The Long Storm* is a fascinating account of Portland during Civil War times. The story also gives a good portrayal of the struggle to control the river freight business.

Nature

The following books are great introductions to the plants and animals that inhabit the wilds of Portland.

A Forest in the City: Your Guide to Tryon Creek State Park. Portland: Friends of Tryon Creek State Park, 1994.

Houle, Marcy Cottrell. *One City's Wilderness: Portland's Forest Park.* Portland: Oregon Historical Society Press, 1987.

Schatz, Jill. C*onifer Tour.* Portland: Hoyt Arboretum, 1990.

Sites and History

Bianco, Joe. *Portland Step-by-Step with Joe Bianco: A Walking Guide to Scenic and Historic Points of Interest.* Beaverton, Ore.: Touchstone Press, 1988.

Klooster, Karl I. *Round the Roses: Portland Past Perspectives. A Collection of Columns Published in "This Week" Magazine Between May 1983 and November 1987.* Portland (PO Box 15173, Portland, 97215), 1987.

Both Bianco and Klooster are former newspapermen. Bianco shares his knowledge as he walks you through the city. Klooster's book consists of reprints of his offbeat columns about quirky happenings in past and present Portland.

O'Donnell, Terence and Thomas Vaughan. *Portland: An Informal History and Guide.* Portland: Oregon Historical Society, 1984.

O'Donnell's graceful prose and thorough research make this an excellent guide to the city.

Snyder, Eugene. *Early Portland: Stump-Town Triumphant.* Portland: Binford and Mort, 1970.

———*Portland: Names and Neighborhoods.* Portland: Binford and Mort, 1979.

———*Portland Potpourri: Art, Fountains and Old Friends.* Portland: Binford and Mort, 1991.

Snyder's accounts of Portland's history are enjoyable, easy to read, and full of interesting anecdotes.

Appendix F: Local Walking Clubs

Portland has many walking groups that are members of the American Volkssport Association. To receive a free general packet that explains volkssports and the American Volkssport Association call the AVA at 1-800-830-WALK and leave your name, address, and telephone number.

Wendy Bumgardner, the current secretary of the AVA, has a fine webpage with many references to articles about walking, as well as lists and links to clubs all over the world. A calendar of events is also available. Check out her page at http://walking.miningco.com. It has everything you would like to know and more.

OTSVA, the Oregon Trail State Volkssport Association is the state chapter of the American Volkssport Association, a network of clubs that sponsor noncompetitive walking, swimming, and hiking events. The following list is of Portland area clubs that sponsor many year-round walks within the city. These walks usually are about 10K (6.2 miles) and can be done at any time of the year.

Columbia River Volkssport Club
1507 A SW Hall
Portland, OR 97201

East County Windwalkers
PO Box 854
Gresham, OR 97030

Lake Oswego Puddle Jumpers
PO Box 1853
Lake Oswego, OR 97035

Rose City Roamers Volkssport Club
6025 N Villard
Portland, OR 97217

Tough Trail Trompers
PO Box 1651
Tualatin, OR 97062

Webfoot Walkers
PO Box 813
Forest Grove, OR 97116

For information on all Oregon walking events, contact OTSVA at 1133 Bexhill, West Linn, OR 97068. OTSVA can give you the local phone numbers for the clubs mentioned above. It also sponsors a Volkssport Information Hotline at 503-620-9098.

Current information on Oregon volkssport events can also be found at http://www.ava.org/walk/or.htm.

Index

Page numbers in *italic* refer to photos.

Meet the Author

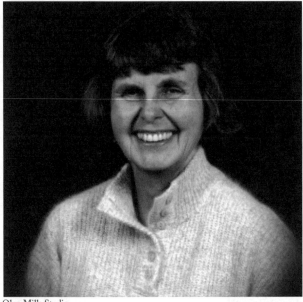

Sybilla Cook grew up in Auburn, New York, and lived in Illinois for 25 years before moving to Oregon. Once in Oregon, her love for the outdoors resurfaced, and she began bicycling, hiking, and walking. She is a member of the Umpqua Valley Walkers, a local chapter of the American Volkssport Association, and has frequently walked the Portland Marathon.

She is a former school library media specialist and consultant for schools in Illinois and Oregon and is the author of *Instructional Design for Libraries,* published by Garland Publishing in 1986, and *Books, Battles, and Bees,* published by the American Library Association in 1994.

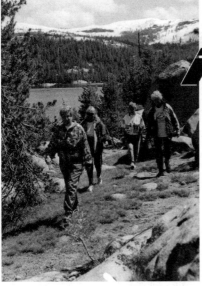 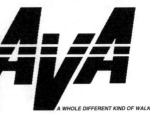

A WHOLE DIFFERENT KIND OF WALK

Experience A Whole Different Kind of Walk

The American Volkssport Association, America's premier walking organization, provides noncompetitive sporting events for outdoor enthusiasts. More than 500 volkssport (translated "sport of the people") clubs sponsor walks in scenic and historic areas nationwide. Earn special awards for your participation.

For a free general information packet, including a listing of clubs in your state, call 1-800-830-WALK. (1-800-830-9255)

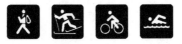

American Volkssport Association is a nonprofit, tax-exempt, national organization dedicated to promoting the benefits of health and physical fitness for people of all ages.

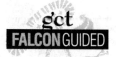

All books in this popular series are regularly updated with accurate information on access, side trips, & safety.

HIKING GUIDES

Hiking Alaska
Hiking Alberta
Hiking Arizona
Hiking Arizona's Catcus Country
Hiking the Beartooths
Hiking Big Bend National Park
Hiking California
Hiking California's Desert Parks
Hiking Carlsbad Caverns &
    Guadalupe Mnts. National Parks
Hiking Colorado
Hiking the Columbia River Gorge
Hiking Florida
Hiking Georgia
Hiking Glacier/Waterton Lakes
Hiking Grand Canyon National Park
Hiking Grand Staircase-Escalante
Hiking Great Basin
Hiking Hot Springs in the Pacific NW
Hiking Idaho
Hiking Maine
Hiking Michigan
Hiking Minnesota
Hiking Montana
Hiking Nevada
Hiking New Hampshire
Hiking New Mexico
Hiking New York
Hiking North Carolina
Hiking North Cascades
Hiking Northern Arizona
Hiking Olympic National Park
Hiking Oregon

Hiking Oregon's Eagle Cap Wilderness
Hiking Oregon's Mt Hood/Badger Creek
Hiking Oregon's Three Sisters Country
Hiking Pennsylvania
Hiking Shenandoah National Park
Hiking South Carolina
Hiking South Dakota's Black Hills Cntry
Hiking Southern New England
Hiking Tennessee
Hiking Texas
Hiking Utah
Hiking Utah's Summits
Hiking Vermont
Hiking Virginia
Hiking Washington
Hiking Wyoming
Hiking Wyoming's Wind River Range
Hiking Yellowstone National Park
Hiking Zion & Bryce Canyon
Exploring Canyonlands & Arches
The Trail Guide to Bob Marshall Cntry

BEST EASY DAY HIKES

Beartooths
Canyonlands & Arches
Glacier & Waterton Lakes
Grand Staircase-Escalante/Glen Cny
Grand Canyon
North Cascades
Olympics
Shenandoah
Yellowstone

FALCON®

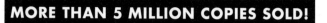

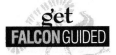

get FALCON GUIDED

MOUNTAIN BIKING GUIDES

Mountain Biking Arizona
Mountain Biking Colorado
Mountain Biking Georgia
Mountain Biking New Mexico
Mountain Biking New York
Mountain Biking N. New England
Mountain Biking Oregon
Mountain Biking South Carolina
Mountain Biking S. New England
Mountain Biking Utah
Mountain Biking Wisconsin

LOCAL CYCLING SERIES

Bend
Boise
Bozeman
Chequamegon
Colorado Springs
Denver/Boulder
Durango
Helena
Moab
White Mountains (West)

BIRDING GUIDES

Birding Minnesota
Birding Montana
Birding Texas
Birding Utah

PADDLING GUIDES

Floater's Guide to Colorado
Paddling Montana
Paddling Okeefenokee
Paddling Oregon
Paddling Yellowstone/Grand Teton

ROCKHOUNDING GUIDES

Rockhounding Arizona
Rockhound's Guide to California
Rockhound's Guide to Colorado
Rockhounding Montana
Rockhounding Nevada
Rockhound's Guide to New Mexico
Rockhounding Texas
Rockhounding Utah
Rockhounding Wyoming

FISHING GUIDES

Fishing Alaska
Fishing Beartooths
Fishing Florida
Fishing Glacier
Fishing Maine
Fishing Montana
Fishing Wyoming
Fishing Yellowstone

■ *To order any of these books, check with your local bookseller
or call The Globe Pequot Press® at **1-800-243-0495**.
Visit us on the world wide web at:*
www.FalconGuide.com

FALCON®

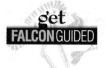

SCENIC DRIVING GUIDES

Scenic Driving Alaska and the Yukon
Scenic Driving Arizona
Scenic Driving the Beartooth Highway
Scenic Driving California
Scenic Driving Colorado
Scenic Driving Florida
Scenic Driving Georgia
Scenic Driving Hawaii
Scenic Driving Idaho
Scenic Driving Michigan
Scenic Driving Minnesota
Scenic Driving Montana
Scenic Driving New England
Scenic Driving New Mexico
Scenic Driving North Carolina
Scenic Driving Oregon
Scenic Driving the Ozarks
Scenic Driving Texas
Scenic Driving Utah
Scenic Driving Washington
Scenic Driving Wisconsin
Scenic Driving Wyoming
Back Country Byways
National Forest Scenic Byways
National Forest Scenic Byways II
Traveling California's Gold Rush Country
Traveling the Lewis & Clark Trail
Traveling the Oregon Trail
Traveler's Guide to the Pony Express Trail

FALCON®

get
FALCON GUIDED

Published in cooperation with Defenders of Wildlife, the Watchable Wildlife® Series is the official series of guidebooks for the National Watchable Wildlife Program. This highly successful program is a unique partnership of state and federal agencies and private organization. Each full-color guidebook in the Watchable Wildlife® series features detailed site descriptions, side trips, viewing tips, and easy-to-follow maps.

WILDLIFE VIEWING GUIDES

Alaska Wildlife Viewing Guide
Arizona Wildlife Viewing Guide
California Wildlife Viewing Guide
Colorado Wildlife Viewing Guide
Florida Wildlife Viewing Guide
Idaho Wildlife Viewing Guide
Indiana Wildlife Veving Guide
Iowa Wildlife Viewing Guide
Kentucky Wildlife Viewing Guide
Massachusetts Wildlife Viewing Guide
Montana Wildlife Viewing Guide
Nebraska Wildlife Viewing Guide
Nevada Wildlife Viewing Guide
New Hampshire Wildlife Viewing Guide
New Jersey Wildlife Viewing Guide

New Mexico Wildlife Viewing Guide
New York Wildlife Viewing Guide
North Carolina Wildlife Viewing Guide
North Dakota Wildlife Viewing Guide
Ohio Wildlife Viewing Guide
Oregon Wildlife Viewing Guide
Tennessee Wildlife Viewing Guide
Texas Wildlife Viewing Guide
Utah Wildlife Viewing Guide
Vermont Wildlife Viewing Guide
Virginia Wildlife Viewing Guide
Washington Wildlife Viewing Guide
West Virginia Wildife Viewing Guide
Wisconsin Wildlife Viewing Guide

- *To order any of these books, check with your local bookseller or call The Globe Pequot Press® at 1-800-243-0495. Visit us on the world wide web at:*
www.FalconGuide.com

FALCON®

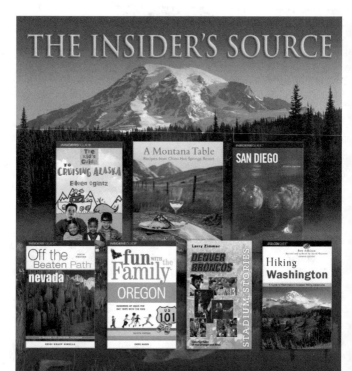
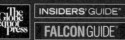